An essay of the great effects
of even languid and unheeded
motion whereunto is annexed An
experimental discourse of some little
observed causes of the insalubrity
and salubrity of the air and its
effects / by Robert Boyle. (1685)

Robert Boyle

An essay of the great effects of even languid and unheeded motion whereunto is annexed An experimental discourse of some little observed causes of the insalubrity and salubrity of the air and its effects / by Robert Boyle.

Boyle, Robert, 1627-1691.

"An experimental discourse of some little observed causes of the insalubrity and salubrity of the air" not present in this copy.

[6], 123 p.

London : Printed by M. Flesher for Richard Davis, 1685.

Wing / B3948

English

Reproduction of the original in the Harvard University Library

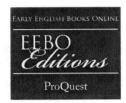

Early English Books Online (EEBO) Editions

Imagine holding history in your hands.

Now you can. Digitally preserved and previously accessible only through libraries as Early English Books Online, this rare material is now available in single print editions. Thousands of books written between 1475 and 1700 and ranging from religion to astronomy, medicine to music, can be delivered to your doorstep in individual volumes of high-quality historical reproductions.

We have been compiling these historic treasures for more than 70 years. Long before such a thing as "digital" even existed, ProQuest founder Eugene Power began the noble task of preserving the British Museum's collection on microfilm. He then sought out other rare and endangered titles, providing unparalleled access to these works and collaborating with the world's top academic institutions to make them widely available for the first time. This project furthers that original vision.

These texts have now made the full journey -- from their original printing-press versions available only in rare-book rooms to online library access to new single volumes made possible by the partnership between artifact preservation and modern printing technology. A portion of the proceeds from every book sold supports the libraries and institutions that made this collection possible, and that still work to preserve these invaluable treasures passed down through time.

This is history, traveling through time since the dawn of printing to your own personal library.

Initial Proquest EEBO Print Editions collections include:

Early Literature

This comprehensive collection begins with the famous Elizabethan Era that saw such literary giants as Chaucer, Shakespeare and Marlowe, as well as the introduction of the sonnet. Traveling through Jacobean and Restoration literature, the highlight of this series is the Pollard and Redgrave 1475-1640 selection of the rarest works from the English Renaissance.

Early Documents of World History

This collection combines early English perspectives on world history with documentation of Parliament records, royal decrees and military documents that reveal the delicate balance of Church and State in early English government. For social historians, almanacs and calendars offer insight into daily life of common citizens. This exhaustively complete series presents a thorough picture of history through the English Civil War.

Historical Almanacs

Historically, almanacs served a variety of purposes from the more practical, such as planting and harvesting crops and plotting nautical routes, to predicting the future through the movements of the stars. This collection provides a wide range of consecutive years of "almanacks" and calendars that depict a vast array of everyday life as it was several hundred years ago.

Early History of Astronomy & Space

Humankind has studied the skies for centuries, seeking to find our place in the universe. Some of the most important discoveries in the field of astronomy were made in these texts recorded by ancient stargazers, but almost as impactful were the perspectives of those who considered their discoveries to be heresy. Any independent astronomer will find this an invaluable collection of titles arguing the truth of the cosmic system.

Early History of Industry & Science

Acting as a kind of historical Wall Street, this collection of industry manuals and records explores the thriving industries of construction; textile, especially wool and linen; salt; livestock; and many more.

Early English Wit, Poetry & Satire

The power of literary device was never more in its prime than during this period of history, where a wide array of political and religious satire mocked the status quo and poetry called humankind to transcend the rigors of daily life through love, God or principle. This series comments on historical patterns of the human condition that are still visible today.

Early English Drama & Theatre

This collection needs no introduction, combining the works of some of the greatest canonical writers of all time, including many plays composed for royalty such as Queen Elizabeth I and King Edward VI. In addition, this series includes history and criticism of drama, as well as examinations of technique.

Early History of Travel & Geography

Offering a fascinating view into the perception of the world during the sixteenth and seventeenth centuries, this collection includes accounts of Columbus's discovery of the Americas and encompasses most of the Age of Discovery, during which Europeans and their descendants intensively explored and mapped the world. This series is a wealth of information from some the most groundbreaking explorers.

Early Fables & Fairy Tales

This series includes many translations, some illustrated, of some of the most well-known mythologies of today, including Aesop's Fables and English fairy tales, as well as many Greek, Latin and even Oriental parables and criticism and interpretation on the subject.

Early Documents of Language & Linguistics

The evolution of English and foreign languages is documented in these original texts studying and recording early philology from the study of a variety of languages including Greek, Latin and Chinese, as well as multilingual volumes, to current slang and obscure words. Translations from Latin, Hebrew and Aramaic, grammar treatises and even dictionaries and guides to translation make this collection rich in cultures from around the world.

Early History of the Law

With extensive collections of land tenure and business law "forms" in Great Britain, this is a comprehensive resource for all kinds of early English legal precedents from feudal to constitutional law, Jewish and Jesuit law, laws about public finance to food supply and forestry, and even "immoral conditions." An abundance of law dictionaries, philosophy and history and criticism completes this series.

Early History of Kings, Queens and Royalty

This collection includes debates on the divine right of kings, royal statutes and proclamations, and political ballads and songs as related to a number of English kings and queens, with notable concentrations on foreign rulers King Louis IX and King Louis XIV of France, and King Philip II of Spain. Writings on ancient rulers and royal tradition focus on Scottish and Roman kings, Cleopatra and the Biblical kings Nebuchadnezzar and Solomon.

Early History of Love, Marriage & Sex

Human relationships intrigued and baffled thinkers and writers well before the postmodern age of psychology and self-help. Now readers can access the insights and intricacies of Anglo-Saxon interactions in sex and love, marriage and politics, and the truth that lies somewhere in between action and thought.

Early History of Medicine, Health & Disease

This series includes fascinating studies on the human brain from as early as the 16th century, as well as early studies on the physiological effects of tobacco use. Anatomy texts, medical treatises and wound treatment are also discussed, revealing the exponential development of medical theory and practice over more than two hundred years.

Early History of Logic, Science and Math

The "hard sciences" developed exponentially during the 16th and 17th centuries, both relying upon centuries of tradition and adding to the foundation of modern application, as is evidenced by this extensive collection. This is a rich collection of practical mathematics as applied to business, carpentry and geography as well as explorations of mathematical instruments and arithmetic; logic and logicians such as Aristotle and Socrates; and a number of scientific disciplines from natural history to physics.

Early History of Military, War and Weaponry

Any professional or amateur student of war will thrill at the untold riches in this collection of war theory and practice in the early Western World. The Age of Discovery and Enlightenment was also a time of great political and religious unrest, revealed in accounts of conflicts such as the Wars of the Roses.

Early History of Food

This collection combines the commercial aspects of food handling, preservation and supply to the more specific aspects of canning and preserving, meat carving, brewing beer and even candy-making with fruits and flowers, with a large resource of cookery and recipe books. Not to be forgotten is a "the great eater of Kent," a study in food habits.

Early History of Religion

From the beginning of recorded history we have looked to the heavens for inspiration and guidance. In these early religious documents, sermons, and pamphlets, we see the spiritual impact on the lives of both royalty and the commoner. We also get insights into a clergy that was growing ever more powerful as a political force. This is one of the world's largest collections of religious works of this type, revealing much about our interpretation of the modern church and spirituality.

Early Social Customs

Social customs, human interaction and leisure are the driving force of any culture. These unique and quirky works give us a glimpse of interesting aspects of day-to-day life as it existed in an earlier time. With books on games, sports, traditions, festivals, and hobbies it is one of the most fascinating collections in the series.

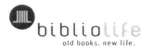

The BiblioLife Network

This project was made possible in part by the BiblioLife Network (BLN), a project aimed at addressing some of the huge challenges facing book preservationists around the world. The BLN includes libraries, library networks, archives, subject matter experts, online communities and library service providers. We believe every book ever published should be available as a high-quality print reproduction; printed on-demand anywhere in the world. This insures the ongoing accessibility of the content and helps generate sustainable revenue for the libraries and organizations that work to preserve these important materials.

The following book is in the "public domain" and represents an authentic reproduction of the text as printed by the original publisher. While we have attempted to accurately maintain the integrity of the original work, there are sometimes problems with the original work or the micro-film from which the books were digitized. This can result in minor errors in reproduction. Possible imperfections include missing and blurred pages, poor pictures, markings and other reproduction issues beyond our control. Because this work is culturally important, we have made it available as part of our commitment to protecting, preserving, and promoting the world's literature.

GUIDE TO FOLD-OUTS MAPS and OVERSIZED IMAGES

The book you are reading was digitized from microfilm captured over the past thirty to forty years. Years after the creation of the original microfilm, the book was converted to digital files and made available in an online database.

In an online database, page images do not need to conform to the size restrictions found in a printed book. When converting these images back into a printed bound book, the page sizes are standardized in ways that maintain the detail of the original. For large images, such as fold-out maps, the original page image is split into two or more pages

Guidelines used to determine how to split the page image follows:

- Some images are split vertically; large images require vertical and horizontal splits.
- For horizontal splits, the content is split left to right.
- For vertical splits, the content is split from top to bottom.
- For both vertical and horizontal splits, the image is processed from top left to bottom right.

AN
ESSAY

Of the Great

EFFECTS

OF

Even Languid and Unheeded

MOTION.

Whereunto is Annexed

An Experimental Difcourfe
of fome little obferved Caufes of the
Infalubrity and Salubrity of the Air
and its Effects.

By the Honourable *ROBERT BOYLE,*
Fellow of the Royal Society.

LONDON,
Printed by *M. Flefher,* for *Richard Davis,*
Bookfeller in *Oxford.* 1685.

ADVERTISEMENT

OF THE

Publisher.

'TIS thought fit the Reader should be in-form'd, That the insuing Tract (about the Effects of Languid Motions) was design'd to be a Part of the Authour's Notes about the Origine of Occult Quali-

ties,

ties, *and ſhould have come*
abroad together with the
Papers about the Effluvia
of Bodies *(moſt of which*
are already publiſh'd.) And
accordingly it was printed
ſeven or eight years ago:
which Circumſtance is here
mention'd, to give a Rea-
ſon why ſeveral Particu-
lars were omitted in the
Body of the Diſcourſe, that
will be found annex'd to the
End of it. For theſe oc-
curring to the Authour
whilſt he curſorily read o-
ver the Tract it ſelf, when

it

it was upon the point to be made publick, 'twas thought fit rather to subjoin them by way of a short Appendix, than to let any thing be lost that seem'd pertinent to so difficult and uncultivated a Subject, as That they belong to. The Reader is farther to be advertis'd, That of the Three Preliminary Discourses, which the Authour intended for *Introductory Ones* to *What* he design'd to say more particularly about the Mechanical Origine or

Pro-

Advertisement of
of Production of Occult
Qualities, One *was con-*
cerning the Relations betwixt the Pores of Bo-
dies and the Figures of
Corpuscles: *but that the*
great Intricacy and Diffi-
culty He found in this co-
pious Subject, made Him
consent, That the Dif-
course of Local Motion,
which should have accom-
pany'd it to the Press *,*
should be printed long before
it. And *those* Papers *about*
Pores and Figures *having*
been for a great while out
of

of the Authour's Power, He now to gratifie the Stationer with something that may in Their stead make up the formerly printed Essay a Book of a convenient Bulk, has put into his Hands what now comes forth, about some Unheeded Causes of the Healthfulness and Insalubrity of the Air: which being chiefly attributed to Subterraneal Steams, Subtile and for the most part Invisible, are as near of kin to the other Effluviums treated of in the Introducto-

ry

ry Discourse, as is requisite
to keep the mention that is
made of them in this Book,
from appearing very incon-
gruous.

A N

AN
ESSAY
Of the Great
EFFECTS
Of
Even *Languid* and *Unheeded*
LOCAL MOTION.

CHAP. I.

HOW superficially soever the *Local Motion* of Bodies is wont to be treated of by the Schools, who admit of divers other Motions, and ascribe almost all strange things in Physicks to *Substantial Forms* and *Real Qualities*; yet it will become Us, who endeavour to resolve the *Phænomena* of Nature into Matter

B   and

and Local motion, (*guided*, at the beginning of things, immediately, and since *regulated*, according to settled Laws, by the Great and Wise Author of the Universe,) to take a heedfull notice of its kinds and operations, as the true Causes of many abstruse Effects. And though the industry of divers late Mathematicians and Philosophers have been very laudably and happily exercised on the nature and general Laws of this Motion; yet I look upon the Subject in its full extent to be of such importance, and so comprehensive, that it can never be too much cultivated, and that it comprises some parts that are yet scarce cultivated at all. And therefore I am not sorry to find my self obliged, by the design of these Notes, (written, as you know, to facilitate the explicating of *Occult* Qualities) to endeavour to improve some neglected Corners of this vast field, and to consider, Whether, besides those effects of Local motion which are more conspicuous, as being produced by the

mani-

manifest striking of one body against another, where the bulk, &c. of the Agent, together with its Celerity, have the chief Interest; there may not be divers effects, wont to be attributed to Occult Qualities, that yet are really produced by *faint* or *unheeded* Local motions of bodies against one another, and that oftentimes at a distance.

But, before I enter upon particulars, this I must premise in general, (which I have elsewhere had occasion to note to other purposes,) that we are not to look upon the bodies we are conversant with, as so many Lumps of Matter, that differ onely in bulk and shape, or that act upon one another merely by their own distinct and particular powers; but rather as bodies of peculiar and differing internal Textures, as well as external Figures: on the account of which structures, many of them must be considered as a kind of Engines, that are both so framed and so placed among other bodies, that sometimes Agents, otherwise in-

B 2   valid,

valid, may have notable operations upon them, becaufe thofe operations being furthered by the Mechanifm of the body wrought on, and the relation which other bodies and Phyfifical Caufes have to it, a great part of the effect is due, not precifely to the external Agent, that 'tis wont to be afcribed to, but in great meafure to the action of one part of the body it felf (that is wrought on) upon another, and affifted by the concurring action of the neighbouring bodies, and perhaps of fome of the more Catholick Agents of Nature. This Notion or Confideration being in other Papers particularly confirmed, I fhall not now infift upon it, trufting that you will not forget it, when there fhall be occafion to apply it in the following Notes.

There may be more Accounts than we have yet thought of, upon which *Local motions* may perform confiderable things, either without being much heeded, or without feeming other then faint, at leaft in relation to

the

the confiderableneſs of the Effects produced by them. And therefore I would not be underſtood in an exclufive ſenſe, when in the following Difcourſe I take notice but of a few of the above-mentioned Accounts; theſe feeming fufficient, whereto, as to Heads, may be conveniently enough referred the Inſtances I allot to this Tract.

And concerning each of theſe Accounts, I hold it requiſite to intimate in this place, that I mention it onely, as that whereon ſuch effects of Local motion, as I refer to it, do principally depend: for, otherwiſe, I am ſo far from denying, that I affert, that in divers caſes there are more Cauſes than one, or perhaps than two of thoſe here treated of apart, that may notably concur to *Phænomena* directly referred to but one or other of them.

To come then cloſer to our ſubject; I ſhall take notice, That among the feverall things, upon whoſe account men are wont to overlook or undervalue the efficacy of Local motions, that are either Unheeded or thought Languid, the chief, or at leaſt thoſe that ſeem to me fitteſt to be treated of in this Paper, are thoſe that are referable to the following Obſervations.

CHAP. II.

Obſervat. I. Men are not uſually aware of the great efficacy of Celerity, even in ſmall Bodies, and eſpecially if they move but through a ſmall ſpace.

WHat a rapid Motion may enable a Body to doe, may be judged by the powerfull and deſtructive Effects of Bullets ſhot out of Cannons, in compariſon of the Battering Engines of the Ancients, which, though I know not how many times bigger then the Bullets of whole Cannon, were not able to batter down Walls and Towers like Bullets, whoſe bulk compared with theirs is inconſiderable. Other examples

of

of a like nature might be without impertinency alledged on this occasion; but, becauſe the latter part of our Propoſition contains that which I chiefly aim at, I ſhall proceed to Inſtances fit to prove That.

I have ſometimes cauſed a skilfull Turner to turn for me an oblong piece of Iron or Steel, and placing my naked hand at a convenient diſtance to receive the little fragments, perhaps for the moſt part leſſer then ſmall pins heads, as they flew off from the rod, they were, as I expected, ſo intenſely heated by the quick action of the Tool upon them, that they ſeemed almoſt like ſo many ſparks of fire; ſo that I could not endure to continue my hand there. And I remember, that once asking an expert workman, whether he (as I had ſometimes done) did not find a troubleſome heat in the little fragments of Braſs that were thrown off when that metall was turning? He told me, that heat was ſometimes very offenſive to his eyes and eye-lids. And

B 4 when

when I asked, whether it was not rather as Duſt caſt into them, than from
their Heat; he replied, that beſides the
ſtroke, he could ſenſibly feel a troubleſome heat, which would make even his
Eye-lids ſore : And that ſometimes,
when he employed a rough Tool, that
took off ſomewhat greater Chips, he
had found the heat ſo vehement, that
not onely 'twould ſcorch his tender
Eye-lids, but the thick and hard skin of
his hands : for proof whereof he
ſhewed me in one of his hands a little
bliſter, that had been ſo raiſed, and
was not yet quite gone off.

And inquiring about theſe matters
of a famous Artiſt, imployed about
the finiſhing up of caſt Ordnance, he
confeſs'd to me, That, when with a
ſtrong as well as peculiar Engine he
and his aſſociates turned great Guns
very ſwiftly, to bring the ſurface to
a competent ſmoothneſs, the tools
would ſometimes throw off bits of metal of a conſiderable bigneſs, which, by
reaſon of their bulk and their rapid
motion, would be ſo heated as to burn
the

the fingers of the Country-people that came to gaze on his work, when he, for merriment fake, defired them to take up fome of thofe pieces of metall from the ground. Which I thought the more remarkable, becaufe by the Contact and Coldnefs of the ground I could not but fuppofe their Heat to have been much allayed. Not to mention, that I learnt from an experienced Artificer, that in turning of Brafs the little fragments of that metall acquire an intenfer Heat than thofe of Iron.

I remember alfo, that, to vary the Experiment mentioned juft before this laft, by making it with a bodie far lefs folid and heavy than Brafs or Iron, I caufed an Artificer to turn very nimbly a piece of ordinary wood, and holding my hand not far off, the powder, that flew about upon the operation, ftruck my hand in many places with that briknefs, that I could but uneafily endure the Heat which they produced where they hit. Which Heat whether it were commumunicated from the little, but much heated, fragments to my hands, or produced there by the brisk percuſſion on my hand, or were the joint effect of both thoſe Cauſes; it will however be a good Inſtance of the power of *Celerity* even in very ſmall bodies, and that move but a very little way.

'Tis conſiderable to our preſent purpoſe, that by an almoſt momentany percuſſion, and that made with no great force, the parts, even of a vegetable, may be not onely intenſely heated, but brought to an actuall Ignition; as we have ſeverall times tried, by ſtriking a good Cane (of that ſort which is fit for ſuch Experiments) with a ſteel, or even with the back of a knife. For, upon this Colliſion, it would ſend forth ſparks of fire like a flint.

To the ſame purpoſe may be alledged, that, by but dextrouſly ſcraping good loaf-ſugar with a knife, there will be made ſo brisk an agitation of the parts, that ſtore of ſparks will

will be produced. But that is more considerable, which happens upon the collision of a flint and a steel : For, though Vitrification be by Chymists esteemed the ultimate action of the fire, and though, to turn sand or stones, though very finely poudered, into glass, 'tis usually required that it be kept for divers hours in the intense fire of a glass-house; and though, lastly, the glass-men complain, that they cannot bring flints or sand to fusion without the help of a good proportion of *Borillia* or some other fixed salt : yet both actuall Ignition and Vitrification are brought to pass almost in a moment by the bare vehemence of that motion that is excited in the parts of a flint when it is struck with a steel: For those sparks that then fly out, (as an Ingenious person has observed, and as I *Mr. Hooke.* have often seen with a good Microscope,) are usually real and permanent parcels (for the most part globulous) of stone vitrified and ignited by the vehemence of the motion. And that
this

this vitrification may be of the stone itself, though steel be a metal of a far more fusible nature then a flint, I am induced to think, because I have tried, that not only flints with steel, but flints with flints, and more easily pieces of Rock-Cryſtal between themſelves, will by colliſion ſtrike fire. And the like effect of colliſion I have found my ſelf in ſome precious ſtones, harder than Cryſtall. And afterwards inquiring of an ingenious Artificer that cuts Diamonds, Whether he had not obſerved the like, when Diamonds were grated on by the rapid motion of his mill? He replied, that he obſerved Diamonds to ſtrike fire almoſt like Flints; which afterwards was confirmed to me by another experienced cutter of Gems; and yet having made divers trials on Diamonds with fire, he would not allow that fire itſelf can bring them to fuſion.

Nor are fluid Bodies, though but of ſmall Dimenſions, to be altogether excluded from the power of making conſiderable impreſſions on ſolid bodies,

bodies, if their celerity be great.

Whether the Sun-beams confift, according to the Atomical Doctrine, of very minute Corpufcles, that, continually iffuing out of the body of the Sun, fwiftly thruft on one another in Phyfically-ftraight Lines; or whether, as the *Cartefians* would have it, thofe beams be made by the brisk action of the Luminary upon the contiguous fluid, and propagated every way in ftraight lines through fome Ethereal matter harboured in the pores of the Air; it will be agreeable to either *Hypothefis*, that the Sun-beams, refracted or reflected by a burning-glafs to a *focus*, do there, by their concourfe, compofe a fmall portion of fluid matter; and yet the *Celerity*, wherewith the foft and yielding fubftance is agitated, enables fo few of them as can be circumfcribed by a Circle, not a quarter of an inch in Diameter, to fet afire green wood in leffe than a minute, and (perhaps in as little time as that) to melt not onely Tinn and Lead thinly

bea-

beaten, but, as I have tried, foliated Silver and Gold.

The operation of small portions of fluid matter on solid bodies will be farther exemplified in the IV. *Chapter*, by the effects of the blown flame of a Lamp on glass and metalls; so that I shall here need but to point in general at the wonderfull effects that *Lightning* has produced, as well by the Celerity of its motion, as by the matter whereof it consists. Of which Effects, Histories and the writings of Meteorologists afford good store; and I have been an admiring observer of some of them, one of the last of which was the melting of metal by the flame in its passage, which probably lasted but the twinckling of an Eye.

And even a small parcel of Air, if put into a sufficiently-brisk motion, may communicate a considerable motion to a solid body; whereof a notable Instance (which depends chiefly upon the Celerity of the springy corpuscles of the Air) is afforded

by

by the violent motion communicated to a bullet fhot out of a good
wind-gun. For, when this Inftrument
is well charged, the ftrongly-compreft
Air being fet at liberty, and forcibly
endeavouring to expand it felf to its
wonted laxity, its corpufcles give a
multitude of impulfes to the bullet,
all the while that it continues moving
along the barrel, and by this means
put it into fo rapid a motion, that I
found by trial, the bullet would in a
moment be flatted, almoft into the
figure of a Hemifphere, by being fhot
off againft a metalline plate.

And farther to fhew, How fwift
that motion muft have been, and with
what Celerity a vehement agitation
may be communicated to the parts of
a Solid body, I fhall add here (though
the *Phænomenon* might be referred to
the V. *Chapter*,) that, though the contact of the Bullet and the metalline
plate lafted probably but a phyfical
moment; yet the minute parts of the
bullet were put into fo various and
brisk an agitation, that making haft

to

to take it up before it should cool,
I found it too hot to be with over-
much ease held between my fingers.

CHAP. III.

Observat. II. *We are too apt to think,
that Fluid bodies, because of their
softness, cannot have by their bare
motion, especially if insensible, any
sensible effect upon Solid ones; though
the fluid moves and acts as an intire
body.*

'TIS not my purpose here to
insist on the efficacy of the
motion of such fluid bodies as may
have their motions discovered by the
eye, like streaming water; or manifestly perceived by the touch, as are
the winds that beat upon us: since
'twere needless to give Instances of
such obvious things, as the great effects of overflowing waters and violent winds; the later of which, notwithstanding the great tenuity and
soft-

softneſs of the air and the *Effluvia* that
ſwim in it, have been ſometimes
able to blow down not onely timber-
trees, but houſes and ſteeples, and o-
ther the firmeſt Structures.   But the
motions I intend to ſpeak of in this
Chapter are ſuch, as we do not immediately either ſee or feel ; and
though theſe be exceeding rare, yet
the operation of *ſounds*, even upon
ſolid bodies, and that at a diſtance
from the ſonorous ones, afford me
ſome Inſtances to my preſent purpoſe,
which I ſhall now proceed to mention.

It has been frequently obſerved,
that, upon the diſcharge of Ordnance
and other great Guns, not onely the
ſound may be diſtinctly heard a great
way off ; but that, to a good diſtance,
the tremulous motion of the Air that
produces ſound, without producing
any ſenſible wind, has been able ſenſibly to ſhake, and ſometimes violently to break, the glaſs-windows of
houſes and other buildings, eſpecially
when the windows ſtand in the way

C   where-

wherein the propagation of the found is directly made. 'Tis true, that these observations are most frequent, when the place, where the Artillery is placed, stands upon the same piece of ground with the Houses whose windows are shaken; and so it may be suspected, that the Shake is first communicated by the Cannon to the earth or floor on which they play, and is afterwards by that propagated through the intermediate parts of the ground to the foundations of the houses, and so to the windows. And I readily grant, and may elsewhere shew, that a violent impulse upon the ground may reach to a greater distance than men usually imagine: But in our present Case I see no necessity of having recourse to any thing but the wave-like motion of the Air for the production of our Phænomenon, since the like may be produced by Local Motion transmitted by Fluids, as may appear by the following Instances.

I was once invited by an Engineer,

to

to fee triall made of a ftrange Inftrument he had to fink fhips, though
great ones, in a few minutes; and
though an unlucky Accident kept
me from arriving there 'till near a
quarter of an hour after the triall had
been made on an old fregat, with better fucceffe than my Philanthropy
allowed me to wifh; yet caufing my
felf to be rowed to the place, where
the great veffell was newly funk,
the odneff of the effect, which was
performed upon the water by a fmall
Inftrument outwardly applied, made
me inquifitive, what noife and commotion had been made: And I was
informed partly by the Engineer himfelf, and partly by fome acquaintances
of mine, who among a great number
of Spectators ftood aloof off in fhips
and other veffels lying at anchor, to
fee the event; that, upon the Engine's operating, the explofion was
fo great, that it made a kind of ftorm
in the water round about, and
did fo rudely fhake veffels that lay at
no inconfiderable diftance, as to make

thofe

thofe that ftood on them to ftagger.

In the late great Sea-fight between the Englifh Fleet commanded by his Royal Highnefs the Duke of *York*, and the Dutch Admiral *Opdam*, (who therein loft the Victory and his Life,) though the Engagement were made very many Leagues from the *Hague*, yet the noife of the Guns not onely reached to that Place, but had a notable effect there; of which when I enquired of the Englifh Embaffadour that as yet refided there, he was pleafed to affure me, that it fhook the windows of his Houfe fo violently, that not knowing what the Caufe was, he was furprized and much alarmed, apprehending, that fome rude Fellows were about to break his windows to affront him. And if there be a greater difpofition in fome other bodies than there is in Glafs-windows to receive ftrong impulfes from the Air agitated by Sounds, thefe may be fenfibly, though not vifibly, wrought upon, and that at a good diftance, by the noife of a fingle

piece

piece of Ordnance ; as may appear
by that memorable Circumſtance of
an odd Caſe about a Gangrene mentioned by the experienced *Simon Pauli*
in his ingenious Tract *de Febribus
malignis*, pag. 71. *Atqui æger ille Gallus
brachio truncatus, octiduum quidem
ſuperfuit, ſed horrendis totius corporis
convulſionibus correptus; qui quoque,
(ut & illa addam obſervatione dig-
niſſima,) dum in Domini ſui ædibus
ad plateam Kiodmoggerianam, Romanè
Laniorum appellares, decumberet, ac,
me ac aliis aliquandiu ad Lectum illius
conſidentibus quidem, ſed nobis non at-
tendentibus, exploderentur tormenta bel-
lica ex Regiis ac Prætoriis navibus, ſi-
niſtrà truncum dextri brachii fovens
ac complectens, toties quoties exploderentur ſingula exclamabat, Au, au, me mi-
ſerum! Jeſu, Maria, contundor penitús:
adeò permoleſta & intolerabilis illi erat
Tormentorum exploſio, & quidem ex
loco ſatis longinquo, terrà non firmà
aut contiguà, verùm ſuper ſalo aut mari
Balthico, inſtituta.* By this it appears,
that the Guns, whoſe diſcharge pro-

C 3   duced

duced thefe painfull motions in the
Patient, refted upon a floating body,
And I remember, that an illuftrious
Commander of a very great Man of
war, being asked by me, whether of
the many wounded men, he had in
his fhip in a very long Sea-fight, none
of them were affected by that noife
of the Enemy's Cannon difcharged in
fhips at a diftance? He anfwered me,
that fome, whofe bones were broken,
would fadly complain of the Tor-
ment they were put into by the fhake
they felt at the going off of the E-
nemy's Cannon, though they were too
much accuftomed to the report of
great Guns, to be, as 'twas a bare
noife, offended by it. If after all
this ti be furmized, that thefe motions
were not conveyed by the air, but
propagated by the water, (and, in
fome cafes, fome part of the fhoar)
from the fhips, where the Guns were
fired, to the Houfes where the windows were fhaken, or the places
where the wounded men lay: I anfwer, that, if this could be made probable,

bable, it would accommodate me with very eminent Inſtances for the Chapter of the *Propagable* nature of Motion : And though it be very difficult to find ſuch examples of ſhakes excited by ſounds as are not liable to the mentioned objection; becauſe the ſonorous bodies here below do all either ſtrike, or lean, upon ſuch groſs and viſible bodies as the Earth and Water ; yet there is one kind of Sound, that muſt be confeſſed to be propagated by the Air , as being made in it; and that is *Thunder*, whoſe noiſe does ſometimes ſo vehemently affect the Air, though without producing any ſenſible wind, that both others and I have obſerved it very ſenſibly to ſhake great and ſtrong Houſes, notwithſtanding the diſtance of the clouds where the noiſes were firſt produced. And I remember, that, having inquired of ſome Sea-Captains, that in ſtout veſſels ſailed to the *Indies*, whether they had nor in thoſe hot Regions obſerved their ſhips, though very much leſs tall then

C 4　　　　houſes,

houſes, to be ſhaken by vehement Thunders? I perceived, that ſome of them had not much heeded any ſuch thing; but a couple of others told me, they had obſerved it in their ſhips; and one of them told me, that once, when the claps of thunder were extraordinary great, ſome of them ſhook his ſhip ſo rudely as to make the unwonted motions diſorder his great Guns. All which I the leſs wonder at, when calling to mind, what I have mention'd in the foregoing Chapter and elſewhere of the power of the Celerity of motion, I conſider, that there is no Celerity that we know of here below, that is near ſo great, as that wherewith a Sound is propagated through the air. For, whereas the diligent *Merſennus* obſerves, that a bullet ſhot out of a Cannon or a Musket does not overpaſs two hundred and forty yards in a Second, or ſixtieth part of a minute; I have more than once diligently obſerved, that the motion of *Sound* paſſes above four hundred yards in the

ſame

same time of a Second here in *England*; which I therefore add, becaufe *Merfennus* relates, that in *France* he obferved a Sound to move in that time many yards more; which may poffibly proceed from the differing confiftence of the Englifh air and the French.

The great Loudnefs of thefe founds, and the vehement percuffion that the Air receives in their formation, will probably make it be eafily granted, that 'twas onely the Impetuofity of the motion of the *Medium*, that gave the fhake to the windows and other folid bodies that I have been mentioning to have been made to tremble by the report of Cannon or Thunder: But yet I will not on this occafion conceal, that perhaps it may without abfurdity be fufpected, that Some of thofe tremulous motions of folid bodies might either depend upon, or at leaft be promoted by, fome peculiar difpofition, that Glaffe (which is endued with fpringinefs,) and fome other bodies that perhaps are not quite devoid of that Quality,

may

may have to be moved by certain congruous Sounds (if I may so call them) more than they would by others, though perchance more loud. But though this surmize should be admitted; yet it would not render the lately-recited Instances improper for the design of this Discourse, but onely would make some of them fit to be referred to another *Chapter*; to which I shall advance, as soon as I shall have annexed an odd Observation of the experienced *Platerus*, which argues, that, where there is a peculiar Disposition, even in a firm body, it may receive considerable impressions from so languid a motion (though in likelihood not peculiarly modified) of the air as is not sensible to other bodies of the same kind.

Plater.Obferv. *Fœmina quædam* (says he)
Lib. 1. p. 185. *in subitaneum incidit morbum, viribus subitò prostratis, se suffocari indesinenter clamitans, etsi nec stertoris nec tussis aliqua essent indicia ; maximè verò de aura quadam adveniente, si vel leviter aliquis adstantium se moveret,*

moveret, quæ illam opprimeret, conque-
rebatur, séque suffocari, si quis propiùs
accederet, clamitabat: vixdum bidu-
um in ea anxietate perseverans, expi-
ravit. To which he adds: *Vidi &*
alios ægros, de simili aura, quæ eos, si quis
illis appropinquaret, in suffocationis pe-
riculum induceret, conquerentes; quod
semper pessimum esse signum depre-
hendi.

CHAP. IV.

Obſervat. III. *Men undervalue the*
motions of bodies too small to be visi-
ble or sensible, notwithstanding their
Numerouſneſs, *which inables them*
to act in swarms.

MOſt men, when they think at all
of the *effluvia* of bodies and their
motions, are wont to think of them as
if they were but much finer ſorts of
Duſt, (whoſe grains, by reaſon of their
ſmalneſs, are inviſible,) which, by
the various agitation of the Air, are

as 'twere by some faint wind blown against the surfaces of the bodies they chance to meet in their way, and that they are stopped in their progress without penetrating into the interior parts of the bodies they invade. And according to this Notion, 'tis no wonder, that men should not fancy, that such minute bodies passing, as they suppose, no further than the surfaces of those on which they operate, should have but faint operations upon them.

But we may have other thoughts, if we well consider, that the Corpuscles we speak of, are, by their minuteness, assisted, and oftentimes by their figure inabled, to pierce into the innermost recesses of the body they invade, and distribute themselves to all, or at least to multitudes of the minute parts, whereof that body consists. For this being granted, though we suppose each single *effluvium* or particle to be very minute ; yet, since we may suppose, even solid bodies to be made up of particles that are so too, and the number of invading particles

to

to be not much inferior to that of the
invaded ones, or at least to be exceedingly great, it need not seem incredi-
ble, that a multitude of little Corpuscles in motion (whose motion, may,
for ought we know, be very swift)
should be able to have a considerable
operation upon particles either qui-
escent, or that have a motion too slow
to be perceptible by sense. Which
may perhaps be the better conceived
by the help of this gross example :
  If you turn an Ant-hill well stoc-
ked with Ants-eggs, upside down,
you may sometimes see such a heap
of eggs mingled with the loose earth,
as a few of those Insects, if they were
yoaked together, would not be able
at once to draw after them ; but if
good numbers of them disperse themselves and range up and down,
and each lay hold of her own egge,
and hurry it away, 'tis somewhat
surprizing to see (as I have with
pleasure done) how quickly the
heap of eggs will be displaced,
when almost every little egge has
one

one of those little Insects to deal
with it.

And in those cases, wherein the invading Fluid does not quite disjoin
and carry off any great number of
the parts of the body it invades, its
operation may be illustrated by that
of the wind upon a tree in *Autumn :*
for, it finds or makes it self multitudes of passages, for the most part
crooked, not onely between the bran-
ches and twigs, but the leaves and
fruits, and in its passing from the
one side to the other of the tree, it
does not onely variously bend the
more flexible boughs and twigs, and
perhaps make them grate upon one
another, but it breaks off some of
the stalks of the fruit, and makes
them fall to the ground, and withall
carries off divers of the leaves, that
grew the least firmly on, and in its
passage does by its differing parts act
upon a multitude of leaves all at
once, and variously alters their si-
tuation.

But to come to closer Instances :
sup-

suppose we cast two lumps, the one
of Sugar, the other of Amber, into a
glass of beer or water, they will both
fall presently to the bottom. And
though perhaps the Amber may be
lighter than the Sugar, (for, I have
found a notable difference in the
specific gravity of pieces of Amber,)
yet the aqueous particles are far
from being able to displace the Amber
or any sensible part of it, or exercise
any visible operation upon it: But
the same minute particles of the li-
quor being of a figure that fits them
to insinuate themselves every way
into the pores of the Sugar, though
the lump consisted of very numerous Saccharine Corpuscles, yet the
multitude of the aqueous particles,
to which they are accessible, is able
in no long time to disperse them all,
and carrying them along with themselves, make the whole lump of Sugar in a short time quite disappear.

The point above discoursed of,
may be more nimbly exemplified in
some Chymical operations, and par-
ticu-

ticularly in this. If, by a due degree
of fire, you abstract from running
Mercury four or five times its weight
of good Oil of Vitriol, there will re-
main at the bottom a dry and brittle
substance exceeding white; and, if
upon this Heap of Mercurial and Sa-
line bodies, which sometimes may be
coherent enough, you pour a good
quantity of limpid water, and shake
them together, you may see in a trice
the multitude of little white grains,
that make up the masse, pervaded,
and manifestly altered, by the dif-
persed Corpuscles of the water ; as
will plainly appear by the change of
the *Calx* or *Precipitate* from a white
masse into one of a fine Limon-co-
lour.

But to give instances in Fluid
bodies, (which I suppose you will
think far the more difficult part of my
task,) though you will easily grant,
that the flame of Spirit of wine, that
will burn all away, is but a visible ag-
gregate of such *Effluvia* swiftly agitated, as without any sensible Heat
would

would of themselves invifibly exhale away; yet, if you be pleafed to hold the blade of a knife, or a thin plate of Copper, but for a very few minutes, in the flame of pure Spirit of wine, you will quickly be able to difcern by the great Heat, that is, the various and vehement agitation of the minute Corpufcles of the metal, what a number of them muft have been fiercely agitated by the pervafion of the igneous particles, if we fuppofe, (what is highly probable,) that they did materially penetrate into the innermoft parts of the metall; and whether we fuppofe this or no, it will, by our experiment, appear, that fo fluid and yielding a body, as the flame of Spirit of wine, is able, almoft in a trice, to act very powerfully upon the hardeft metalls.

The power of extreamly-minute parts of a fluid body, even when but in a moderate number they are determined to confpire to the fame operation, may be eftimated by the

D   moti-

motions of Animals, especially of the larger and more bulky sorts, as Horses, Bulls, Rhinocerots and Elephants. For, though the animal spirits be minute enough to be invisible, and to flow through such tender passages, that prying Anatomists have not been able in dissected Nerves to discern so much as the channels through which they pass; yet those Invisible Spirits, conveyed (or impelled) from the Brain to the Nerves, serve to move in various manners the Lims, and even the unwieldy bodies themselves of the greatest Animals, and to carry them on in a progressive motion for many hours together, and perhaps enable them to spring into the Air, and move through it by leaping; though divers of these Animals weigh many hundred, and others several thousand of pounds.

I will not here consider, whether the following Experiment may at all illustrate Motions that are produced by the fluid parts of Animals in some

of the confiftent ones : But I prefume, it may confirm the Obfervation
maintained in this Chapter, if I add,
what I have tried of the confiderable
force of a number of aqueous particles,
as flexible and as languid as they are
thought to be, infinuating themfelves
into the pores or Intervals of a rope
that was not thick. For in moift
weather I fometimes obferved, that
the aqueous and other humid particles, fwimming in the air, entering the
pores of the hemp in great numbers,
were able to make it fhrink, though
a weight of fifty, fixty, or even
more pounds of lead were tied at the
end to hinder its contraction, as appeared by the weights vifibly being
raifed in wet weather above the
place it refted at in dry.

But to return to what I was formerly fpeaking of the Determinati-
on of the motion of Fluids; I fhall,
on this occafion, obferve, that, though
the wind or breath, that is blown
out at a fmall crooked pipe of metal
or glafs, fuch as Tradesmen for its

D 2 ufe

use call a Blow-pipe, seems not to have any great celerity, especially in comparison of that of the parts of flame; and is it self of little force; yet, when by this wind the flame of a Lamp or Candle is directed so as to beat with its point upon a body held at a convenient distance from the side of the flame, the burning fluid, determined, and perhaps excited by this wind, acquires so great a force, that, as we have often tried, it may be made, in a few minutes, to melt not onely the more fusible Metals, but silver, or even copper it self; which yet may be kept for many hours unmelted in a Crucible kept red-hot, or even in the flame of the Lamp or Candle, unassisted by the blast.

And if we can so contrive it, that a flame does not come to invade onely the surface that invests a body, but comes to be intermingled with the smaller (though not the smallest) parts it consists of, as with its filings or its powder; the flame will then have a far more quick and powerfull

ope-

operation than the body expofed to it. This I exemplify (in other Papers) and in this place it may fuffice to obferve, that, whereas a pound or two of Tartar may coft you fome hours to calcine it to whitenefs, if the flame have immediate accefs onely to the outward parts; you may calcine it in a very fmall part of that time, if, mixing with its grofs powder an equal weight of good Salt-peter, you fire the mixture, and keep it ftirring, that the parts of the kindled Nitre may have accefs at once to very many parts of the Tartar, and have opportunity to calcine them. And by fomewhat a like artifice, I elfe-where teach, how Nitre it felf may without Tartar be fpeedily reduced to a *Calcinatum*, not unlike that newly mentioned. But it may be faid, that fome of the foregoing Inftances (for it cannot be truly faid of all) may indeed illuftrate what we are dif-courfing of, but will not reach home to our purpofe.

I fhall therefore confider the

D 3   *Load-*

Load-stone, which you acknowledge to act by the emission of Insensible particles. For, though Iron and Steel be solid and ponderous bodies, and Magnetical *effluvia* be corpuscles so very minute, that they readily get in at the pores of all kind of bodies, and even of Glass it self; yet these Magnetical *effluvia*, entring the steel in swarms, do in a trice pervade it, and a multitude even of Them, acting upon the Corpuscles of the metal, do operate so violently on them, that, if the *Load-stone* be vigorous enough, and well capped, it will attract a notable proportion of steel, and surmount the gravity of that solid metal, which I have found to exceed, when the stone has been very good and little, above fifty times the weight of the Magnet by whose *effluvia* it was supported: For, to these I rather ascribe Magnetical attraction and sustentation, than to the impulse or pressure of the ambient air, to which many Corpuscularians have recourse; because I have found by trial (which

I else-

I elsewhere relate) that the pressure of the ambient air is not absolutely necessary to Magnetical operations.

I remember, that, to help some friends to conceive, how such extreamly-minute particles as Magnetical *effluvia*, may, by pervading a hard and solid body, such as Iron, put its insensible Corpuscles into motion, and thereby range them in a new manner, I took filings of Steel or Iron freshly made, that the Magnetical virtue might not be diminished by any rust, and having laid them in a little heap upon a piece of paper held level, I applied to the lower side of the paper, just beneath the Heap, the pole of a vigorous Load-stone, whose Emissions traversing the paper, and diffusing themselves through the incumbent metall, did in a trice manifestly alter the appearance of the Heap ; and, though each of the filings might probably contain a multitude of such small Martiall Corpuscles as Steel may be divided into by Oil of Vitriol or Spirit of Salt ; yet the Mag-

neti-

netical *effluvia*, immediately pervading our metalline heap, did so remove a good part of the filings that composed it, as to produce many erected aggregates, each of which consisted of several filings placed one above another, and appearing like little needles, or rather like the ends of needles broken off at some distance from the point. And as these little temporary needles stood all of them erected (though more or less, according to their distance from the Pole of the Magnet) upon the flat paper; so they would, without losing their figure or connexion, be made as it were to run to and fro upon the paper, according as the Load-stone, that was held underneath it, was moved this way and that way; and as soon as that was taken quite away, all this little stand of pikes (if I may so call it) would (almost in the twinkling of an eye) relapse into a confused heap of filings.

There are two ways of explicating the turning of Water into Ice; one

of

or other of which is approved almost
by all the Corpuscularian Philosophers. The first is that of the *Cartesians*, who give an account of Glaciation by the recesse of the less subtile
particles of the Etherial matter,
without which the finer parts were
too small and feeble to keep the Eel-
like particles of water flexible, and
in the form of a liquour. The *Atomists* on the other side ascribe the freezing of water to the ingress of multitudes of *frigorifick* Corpuscles,
as they call them, which, entering
the water in swarms, and dispersing
themselves through it, crowd into
the pores, and hinder the wonted motion of its parts, wedging themselves
(if I may so speak) together with
them into a compact body. But
which soever of these two *Hypothe-
ses* be pitched upon, the Phænomenon it self will afford me a notable
Instance to my present purpose. For,
the Particles of water, and much
more the Corpuscles of cold, are confessed to be singly too small to be
visible,

visible, and their motions are not said to be swift, but may rather be judged to be slow enough ; and yet those minute aqueous, or more minute frigorifick particles, because of their number, produce in the glaciation of the liquour so forcible a motion outwards, as to make it break bottles, not onely of glass and earth strongly baked, but, as I have several times tried, of metal it self, that being full of the liquour were firmly stopped before the supervening of the Cold. And the expansive endeavour of freezing water is not onely capable of doing this, but of performing so much greater things, which I elsewhere relate, that my trials have made me sometimes doubt, whether we know any thing in nature, except kindled Gunpowder, that bulk for bulk moves more forcibly, though the motion seems to be very slow.

CHAP.

CHAP. V.

(Of the Propagable Nature of Motion.)

Obfervat. IV. *Men are not fufficient-*
ly aware, how propagable Local Mo-
tion is, even through differing Medi-
ums, and Solid bodies.

THere are four principal Occa-
fions on which I have obferved, that men are wont to think the
Communicating of Motion much
more difficult than indeed it is.

And *firft,* there are many, that obferving how ufually thofe bodies
that hit againft hard ones rebound
from them, eafily perfwade themfelves, that Motion can fcarce be
tranfmitted or diffufed through Solid
bodies. But though it be true, that
oftentimes in fuch cafes the pro-
greffive motion of the body or the

Solid,

Solid, that is ſtruck or impelled, be
either inconſiderable, or, perhaps, not
ſo much as ſenſible; yet the impulſe
may make a conſiderable impreſſion,
and may be communicated to a great
ſhare of the particles of that matter,
whereof the ſolid maſs conſiſts; as we
ſee in the ſtriking of a timber-beam at
one end, the motion, though perhaps
it were not ſtrong at the firſt, may
become ſenſible at the other. Though
Bell-metal be ſo hard a body, that it
is reckoned harder than iron it-ſelf,
inſomuch that oftentimes it reſiſts
even files of Steel, which readily
work on Iron; yet this ſolidity hin-
ders not but that, as I have found,
conveniently ſhaped veſſels of Bell-
metal, though thick, will be ſenſibly
affected by a motion that neither
is ſtrong, nor touches them in
more than a ſhort line, or perhaps
than a Phyſical point.   The truth of
this I have found by trial on more
than one ſuch veſſels and particularly
on one that was hemiſphærical, which
being placed or held in a convenient
poſture,

posture, if I did but gently pass the point of a pin for a little way along the brim of it, it would sensibly resound, and that (to a very attentive ear) so long, and in such a ringing manner, as made it highly probable, that the parts, immediately touched (and not so much as scratched)by the point of a pin, were not onely put into a vibrating motion themselves, but were enabled to communicate it to those that were next them, and they to those that were contiguous to them; and so the tremulous motion was propagated quite round the bell, and made divers successive Circulations before it quite ceased to be audible. And if, in stead of drawing a Line on the brim of the vessel, I struck it, though but faintly, with the point of a pin, though the part immediately touched would be but a physical point, yet the motion would be, like the former, propagated several times quite round; as was argued by the ringing and duration of the produced sound, though this

metal-

metalline veffel were feven inches
in Diameter, and of a confiderable
thicknefs. Nor was a folidity like
that of Brafs requifite to produce
thefe effects. For I found them to
infue much after the fame manner,
when I employed onely a fhort and
flender thread of Glafs, which though
little, if at all, thicker than a pin, was
yet hollow quite through. Now
if it be true, as 'tis highly probable,
that Sound, as it belongs to the air,
confifts in an undulating motion of
the Air, and fo in our cafe requires
a vibrating motion in the fonorous
body to impart that motion to the
Air; we muft grant in our Inftances
a wonderfull propagablenefs of motion, even when 'tis not violent, in
Solid bodies themfelves; fince the
point of a pin, gently ftriking a part,
no bigger than it felf, of a mafs of very
folid metal, could thereby communicate a fenfible motion, and that feveral times circulated, to millions of
parts equall to it in bulk, and much
exceeding it in hardnefs. And fince
the

the effect was more confiderable, when the trial was made in a much greater, than in a fmaller veffel; 'tis probable, that, if I had had the opportunity of experimenting on a large and well-hung Bell, the *Phænomenon* would have been more notable; as it alfo feemed to be on our veffel, if, in ftead of ftriking it with the point of a pin, we caft, though but faintly, againft the lower part of it a grain of fhot, lefs than a fmall pins-head, or let a little grain fall, from about one foot high, upon the infide of the inverted Hemifphere. And to fhew, that even foft and yielding bodies, and but faintly moved, are not to be excluded from a power of putting fuch hard ones into motion; I fhall add, that I found almoft the like effects to thofe above mentioned, by paffing the pulp of my finger a little way along the lower part of the veffel. Nay, that fluid bodies themfelves may communicate fuch an inteftine and propagable motion, to harden folid ones, I may have hereafter

after an occasion to shew by the
effects of a small Flame, and the
Sun-beams on glass and steel. And
I shall here on this occasion add
this word about the Propagation of
Motion produced in solid bodies by
heat, that it much depends upon the
particular Textures of the bodies.
For I found, that when I heated a
piece of glass or of a fire-stone, I could
without inconvenience hold my naked hand upon parts that were very
near (suppose within an inch off) the
ignited portions of them. But, if we
take a rod of Iron, for instance, and
heat one end red-hot, the heat of that
end will be so propagated towards
the other, that it will offend one's
hand at several times the distance,
at which one might conveniently
hold the rod, if it were of glass.

In many buildings it may be observed, (and is thought a sign of the firm
Cohesion of their parts,) that a
stamp of one's foot, nay or bare
treading, or some such other lesse
brisk impulse, made in one room,
will

will have a fenfible effect in all or moft of the others. And it often happens, that, by the hafty fhutting of a door, the whole houfe is made to tremble; whence we may argue, that, even among folid bodies, motion made in one place may be readily propagated to many others: And if, as to the latter of the Inftances, the fudden impulfe and compreffion of the Air, made by the door fuppofed to be haftily fhut, have any confiderable fhare in the effect, the Phænomenon will ferve to fhew the efficacy even of fuch a motion of a fluid body, as we cannot directly feel upon divers large and firmly connected folid bodies.

In *Earthquakes* the tremulous motion fometimes extends fo very far, that, though it feems highly probable, that the fhake that is given to one part of the Earth by the firing and explofion of fubterraneal exhalations, (if that be the true and onely caufe of Earthquakes) is not capable of reaching near fo far as divers

E Earth-

Earthquakes have done, but that the fire paſſes through ſome little ſubterraneal clefts, or channels, or hidden conveyances, from one great Cavity or Mine to another; yet 'tis not improbable but that the vehemently tremulous motion does oftentimes reach a very great way beyond the places where the exploſions were made. Since, though *Seneca* would confine the extent of Earthquakes to two hundred miles, yet obſervations made in this and the laſt Century warrant us to allow them a far greater ſpread. The Learned *Joſephus Acoſta* affirms, that in the Kingdom of *Peru* in the year 1586 an Earthquake reached along the ſhoar of the Pacifick ſea 160 Leagues; and adds, that ſometimes it has in thoſe parts run on from South to North 300 Leagues. And in the beginning of this our age (*Anno Dom.* 1601) good writers relate a much larger Earthquake to have happened, ſince it reached from

Natur. Quæſt. Lib. VI. Cap. 25.

Lib. III. Cap. 26.

Aſia

Asia to that Sea that washes the *French* Shoars, and, besides some *Asiatick* Regions, shook *Hungary, Germany, Italy* and *France,* and consequently a great part of *Europe.* And if that part of the Narrative be certain, which relates, that this lasted not much above a quarter of an hour, it will be the more likely, that this Earthquake shook great Tracts of Land beyond those places, to which the fired matter, passing from one cavity to another, could reach in so short a time: As you will the more easily guesse, if you try, as I have done, that in trains of Gunpowder it self the fire does not run on near so swiftly as one would imagine. But though I have been in more Earthquakes then one; yet, since they were too sudden and too short to afford me any considerable observation, I shall say no more of them; but proceed to take notice, that oftentimes the motion of a Coach or Cart, that passed at a good distance from the place that I was in, has made the

buildings

buildings fo fenfibly fhake, that I
could not but wonder, that fo great a
portion of fo firm and fluggifh a body, as the Earth, could, by a caufe
that feemed very difproportionate to
fuch an effect, be made to tremble
it felf, and manifeftly to fhake firm
buildings that were founded on it.
And this obfervation made me the
more inclinable to give credit to their
Relations, who tell us, that in a calm
night, the march of a troup of horfe
may be felt, by attentive Scouts
watching at a great diftance off, by
the fhake that the ground receives
from the trampling of the horfes;
though I formerly fufpected much,
and do yet a little, that the impulfe
of the air conveyed along the refifting
furface of the ground, might mainly
contribute to the effect that is afcribed onely to the motion of the foil.

Before I advance to the *Second*
Member of this Chapter, it may not
be impertinent to note, that in peculiarly difpofed bodies, and efpecially
in Organical ones, a very *languid*
moti-

motion may have a far greater effect, than it could produce by a bare propagation of it self. For it may so determine the motion of the Spirits or other active parts of the body it works on, as to make multitudes of them act as if they conspired to perform the same motions. As when a ticklish man, by having the pulp of one's finger passed gently along the sole of his foot or the palm of his hand, has divers muscles and other parts of his body and face put into preternatural or unusual motions. And most men by being lightly tickled with the end of a feather or straw, within their Nostrils, have their heads and many parts of their bodies put into that violent Commotion, wherein *Sneezing* consists. And I remember, that having for some time been, by a distemper, (from which God was graciously pleased a while after to free me,) quite deprived of the use of my hands; it more than once hapned to me, that sitting alone in a Coach, if the wind chanced to

blow

blow a single hair upon my face in the Summer-time, the tickling or itching, that it produced, was so uneasy to me, 'till by calling out to a footman I could get it removed, that, though I could well bear it as long as I was wont to do, when, having the use of my hands, I could relieve my self at pleasure; yet if I were forced to endure the itching too long, before any came to succour me, the uneasiness was so great, as to make me apprehend falling presently either into Convulsions or a Swoon. But 'tis time to proceed to the *second* Member of this Chapter.

2. Others there are, that cannot believe, that Local motion, especially if it be *languid,* can be propagated through differing Mediums, each of which, save that wherein the Motion is begun, must, they think, either repell, or check and dead it. To these I shall recommend the Consideration of an Experiment, I remember I made before some Learned men in our Pneumatick Engine. For, having

cau-

caufed a large and thick glafs Receiver to be fo blown, that it had a
glafs button in the infide of that part
which upon the Engine was to be
placed upwards; I caufed a Watch
to be fufpended by a little Silver-
chain faftned to that button by as
flender and foft a body, as I thought
would be ftrong enough to fupport
my watch; and then, the Glafs being
cemented on clofe to the Receiver,
to prevent a Commerce between the
Cavity of it and the Air, the watch,
that hung freely near the middle of
the Cavity of the Receiver, made it
felf to be heard by thofe attentive
Liftners, that would hold their ears
directly over the fufpended watch,
whofe motions were thereby argued
to have been propagated, either
through the included air, or along the
ftring to the concave part of the
Glafs, and through the whole thicknefs of the Glafs to the convex part,
and thence, through the interpofed
air to the Ear. And this mention of
watches minds me of what I often ob-

ferved

served in a fmall ftriking watch, that
I have worn in my pocket. For,
when it ftruck the Hours, and in fome
poftures when the balance did but
move, I could plainly feel the brisker
motions of the Bell, and fenfibly the
languid ones of the balance, through
the feveral linings of my Breeches,
and fome other interpofed foft and
yielding bodies; and this, though
the watch (as I faid) was fmall, and
the balance included in a double cafe,
and though the outwardmoft were
of (what they call) Chagrine, and
the innermoft of Gold; which I therefore mention, becaufe that clofeft of
metals is obferved more to dead
founds and motions than harder metals, as Silver, Copper, and Iron.

That Motion may be propagated
through differing Mediums, may feem
the more probable by the fhakings
that are often felt by men lying on
beds that ftand in rooms clofe fhut,
when loud claps of thunder are produced (perhaps at a great diftance
off) in the clouds. And whether it
will

will be fit to add to this Instanc^e
that which you have lately met with
in the III. Chapter of a wounded
Frenchman at *Copenhagen*, I leave you
to confider.

I know not whether it will be very
proper to take notice on this occafion of an odd *Phænomenon* recited by
the experienced *Agricola*
in thefe words. *Si animal
dejicitur in antrum Vi-
burgenfe, quod eft in Carelia, Regione
Scandiæ, erumpit, ut perhibent, fonus
intolerabilis magno cum flatu: Si leve
pondus in fpecum Dalmatiæ, quamvis,
inquit Plinius, tranquillo die, turbini
fimilis emicat procella.*

*De nat. eorum
quæ eft. è Terra
Lib. IV. Cap. 7.*

3. As thofe of whom I took notice at the beginning of this Chapter,
are backward to allow, that Motion
may be confiderably propagated
through *folid* bodies; fo on the con-
trary, there are others that are indifpofed to think, that 'tis near fo propagable as indeed it is through *fluid*
bodies; becaufe they prefume, that
the eafy ceffion of the parts of fluids
will

will dead the impulse received by thofe of them that are firft acted on by the impelling body. And

4. There is yet another fort of Naturalifts, who, though they may be brought to grant, that Motion may by propagated even through a foft and yielding Medium, cannot believe, that it fhould through fuch a Medium be propagated to any confiderable diftance; being perhaps induced to this opinion by obferving, that, though a body fomewhat broad as well as folid, as the Palm of one's hand or a battledore, be moved through the Air fwiftly enough to make a wind; yet that wind will not be ftrong enough to be felt any more than a very little way off. Wherefore, becaufe the Inftances, to which I affign the remaining part of this Chapter, may be for the moft part applicable to the removal of both thefe prejudices; It may for brevity fake be expedient to confider them both together.

If Luminous bodies act on our Eyes,

Eyes, not by a substantial diffusion
of extreamly minute particles, as the
Atomists would have it, but by a propagated Pulsion of some Subtile matter contiguous to the shining body,
(as the *Cartesians* and many other
Philosophers maintain;) 'twill be manifest, that a body less than a small
pin's head may give a brisk motion to
a portion of fluid matter many millions of times greater than it self;
since in a dark night a single spark of
fire may be seen in differing places,
whose distance from it exceeds many thousand times the spark's *Diameter.* Not to mention the great
remove, at which the flame of a small
taper may not onely be seen, but appear greater than near at hand. And
if we compare the *Diameter* of that
bright Planet *Venus*, which yet
shines but with a borrowed and reflected Light, with its *distance* from
the Earth, we may easily conclude,
that the fixed Stars, which probably
are so many Suns that shine by their
own native Light, must impell a stu-
pendi-

pendious proportion of Etherial matter, to be able at that immense distance to make such vivid Impressions, as they do, upon our Eyes. But to descend to Instances less remote and disputable, I shall, in order to the removal of the two lately mentioned prejudices, proceed to consider; that, though it be true, that Fluid bodies do easily yield to Solid ones that impell them, and thereby oftentimes quickly dead the motion of those Solids; yet the motion, being lost onely in regard of the solid body, is not lost, but transmitted and diffused in reference to the fluid. As when a log of wood, or any such body specifically lighter than water, is let fall in the middle of a pond, though its progress downwards be checkt, and it be brought to rest quietly on the surface of the water; yet its motion is not lost, but communicated to the parts of the water it first strikes against, and by those to others, till at length the curls or waves produced on the surface of the water
water

ter spread themselves, till they arrive
at the brinks, and would perhaps be
farther expanded, if these did not
hinder their progress. From which
inftance we may learn, that, though
the nature of fluid bodies, as fuch, requires, that their parts be actually
diftinct and feparately moved; yet
the particular Corpufcles that compofe them, being (at leaft here below) touched by divers others, the
new motion that is produced in fome
of them by an impellent Solid, muft
needs make them impell the contiguous Corpufcles, and thefe thofe that
chance to lie next to them, and fo the
impulfe may be propagated to a diftance; which you will the more eafily believe may be great, if you confider with me, both that in a fluid
body the Corpufcles, being already
in the various motion requifite to
fluidity, yield more eafily to the impellent, and alfo that being fully, or
very near it, counterpoifed by others
of the fame fluid, a fcarce imagina-
bly little force may fuffice to impell
them;

them; infomuch that, though the brafs Scale of a balance, of divers inches in Diameter, may well be fuppofed to outweigh many myriads of fuch particles as compofe water, wine, &c. yet, (as I elfewhere more fully relate) when fuch a fcale was duly counterpoifed with another like it, I could eafily put it into various motions onely with the invifible *Effluvia* of no great piece of Amber. And if we confider that obvious Inftance of the fwelling Circles made by cafting a ftone into a Pond or other ftagnant water, we fhall be the more eafily perfwaded, that, even in a heavy fluid, a motion may reach a far greater way, than men are ufually aware of, beyond the parts on which it was firft impreft.

On this occafion I muft not omit a ftrange Obfervation given me by a very experienced Navigator, that much frequents the Coaft of *Groenland*, and other *Arctick* Regions, to fifh for whales. For this perfon being difcourfed with by me about the ef-
feéts

fects of the breaking of thofe vaft piles of Ice, that are to be met with in thofe parts, affured me, that not onely he had often heard the Ice make in breaking terribler noife than the loudeft claps of thunder with us, but that fometimes, when the Sea-water had, as it were, undermined the foundation of the mountainous piece of Ice, he has known it at length fuddenly fall into the fubjacent Sea with fo much violence as to make a ftorm at a great diftance off ; infomuch that once, when he lay two Leagues off of the place where this ftupendious mafs of Ice fell, it made the waves goe fo high as to wafh clear over the ftern of the fhip, with danger enough to fome of his men, and to fink feveral of his fhallops that were riding by, though fcarce any fmall veffels in the world ufe to be fo fitted for rough Seas as thofe about *Groenland.*

And whereas, though the Air be a much thinner fluid, we are apt to think it indifpofed to propagate mo-

tion

tion far, give me leave to tell you, that we may take wrong meafures, if we think, that, (for inftance) the undulating motion, into which the Air is put by the action of fonorous bodies, reaches but a little way, as we are apt to prefume it does, becaufe we judge of it by the effect it has on our ears when the found is made in difadvantageous places. For one, that, for inftance, hears a Lute or a Viol plaid on in a room furnifhed with hangings, will be apt to think the found faint and languid in comparifon of what it would appear to him, if the fame Inftrument were plaid on after the fame manner in an arched room without hangings; thefe foft and yielding bodies being apt to dead the found, which the figure and hardnefs of the Vaulted room would reflect. And fo, when a man fpeaks aloud in the free Air, we are not wont to take any notice of a progrefs made by the motion of the Air beyond the place we are in, when our ears receive the found; but if the place happen

to

to be furnished with an *Echo*, though at many times that diftance from the fpeaker, we may then eafily take notice, that the motion of the Air was carried on, and that with good vigour, to a far greater diftance than elfe we fhould have obferved. And I have often thought, that, even by the better fort of our Echoing places, we are not informed, to near how great a fphere the motion, which the Air is put into by Sounds, may extend it felf, where its diffufion and vigour are not hindred nor weakned by bodies either placed too near, or indifpofed to promote its operation.

What has been lately faid of the great diffufion of Sounds, if themfelves be loud and great, will appear highly probable, by what is related by the Learned *Fromundus*, who being Profeffour of Philofophy at *Lovain*, in the Year 1627, had opportunity enough to know the Truth of what he relates; namely that, at the famous Siege of *Oſtend* in *Flanders*, the

From. Meteor. Lib. II. Art. 9.

F   thun-

thunder of the great Ordnance was heard at above thirty Dutch Leagues, which, according to the vulgar reckoning, amounts to a hundred and twenty of our English miles. And that is yet, as he truly obſerves, more ſtrange, and makes more for our preſent purpoſe, which he adds concerning the diffuſion of the ſound of a Drum, which, he ſays, was, upon a time, heard at Sea twelve Leagues off.

But to return to what I was ſaying of *Echo's*, to confirm my conjecture about them, I ſhall think it needleſſe to offer you any other Argument, than that which you will draw your ſelf from the Notable Relation I met with in the Learned *Va-*

Geograph. general. Lib. I. Cap. XIX.

renius of an Obſervation made by *David Frælichi-us*, who, in the Company of a couple of Students, had the curioſity (in the month of *June*) to viſit the mountain *Carpathus*, eſteemed the higheſt of all the *Hungarian* Hills, and ſaid to be much more ſteep and difficultly acceſcessible than any of the *Alps* themselves. *Frælichius* then (in my Authour) having related with what difficulty he and his Companions ascended above that Region of the Air, where they met with clouds and vehement winds, adds this memorable Observation, for whose sake I mention the story : *Exploss* (saies he) *in ea summitate sclopetum, quod non majorem sonitum primò præ se tulit, quàm si tigillum vel bacillum confregissem ; post intervallum autem temporis murmur prolixum invaluit, inferiorésque montis partes, convalles, & sylvas opplevit. Descendendo per nives annosas intra convalles, cùm iterum sclopetum exonerarem, major & horribilior fragor quàm ex tormento capacissimo inde exoriebatur : hinc verebar, nè totus mons concussus mecum corrueret ; duravitque hic sonus per semiquadrantem horæ, usque dum abstrusissimas cavernas penetrasset, ad quas Aer undique multiplicatus resiliit. Et talia quidem objecta concava in summitate se non illico offerebant, idcirco ferè insensibiliter*

primùm

*primùm sonus repercutiebatur, donec
descendendo antris & convallibus vi-
cinior factus, ad eas fortiùs impegit.*

CHAP. VI.

Observat. V. *Men usually think not
what the modification of the invisible motion of Fluids may perform on
the disposed bodies of Animals.*

IN this Observation I expresly mention *the disposed bodies of Animals*, to intimate, that there is a peculiar aptitude required in those Animals,
or some particular parts of them that
are to be sensibly affected by such
motions as we are treating of, which
would otherwise be too languid to
have any sensible operation on
them.

It seems the less strange to me, that
continuing Sounds, and other somewhat durable Impulses of the Air or o-
ther Fluids, should have a manifest operation upon Solid bodies, when I consider

der the multitude of strokes that may in a very short and perhaps scarce observable time, be supposed to be given by the parts of the fluid to the Consistent body. For, though each of these single would perhaps be too languid to have any sensible effect at all; it being opportunely and frequently repeated by the successive parts of the fluid, as by so many little swimming hammers or flying bullets, they may well have a notable effect upon the parts of a body exposed to their action: As may be argued from the great swing that may be given to Pendulums by a very languid force, if it successively strike the swinging body, when having finished its excursion, 'tis ready to return towards the Perpendicular; as also from the tremulous motion that is imparted even to the metalline string of a Musical Instrument, by the congruous motion the Air is put into by another trembling string, (as there may be hereafter occasion to declare.)

I remember, *Scaliger* tells a plea-

sant

fant story of a Knight of *Gascony*, whom the found of a Bagpipe would force prefently to make water ; adding, that a Perfon difobliged by this man, and refolving to be merrily revenged on him, watched a time when he fate at a Feaft fo as he could not well get out, and brought a Bagpiper to play unawares behind him ; which he did fo unluckily, that the Mufick had prefently its wonted effect upon the poor Knight, to his great Confufion and the laughter of the Company. On which occafion I fhall add, that I know a very Ingenious Gentleman, who has confeffed to me, that the noife of a running Tap is wont to have almoft the like operation upon Him.

'Tis a common Obfervation, that the noife that an ungreafed cartwheel makes in grating againft the axel-tree, and the fcraping of a knife upon a plate of filver or pewter, and fome other fuch brisk and acute Sounds, do fo affect divers parts of the Head, as to produce that effect

that

that is commonly called *setting the Teeth on edge* ; which whether it proceed from any commerce between the Auditory Nerves, and those that are inservient to the motion we have mentioned, I leave Anatomists to consider. But these effects of acute sounds are much less considerable than that which I elsewhere relate of an Ingenious Domestick of mine, who several times complained, that the tearing of brown paper made his Gums bleed : which argued that the sound had an operation not onely upon the nervous and membranous parts, but the bloud and Humours themselves.

Sir *Henry Blunt*, in his voiage to the *Levant*, giving an account of what he observed in *Egypt*, has, among other remarkable things, this passage : Many rarities of Living creatures I saw in *Gran Cairo*, but the most ingenious was a nest of four-legged Serpents of two foot long, black and ugly, kept by a Frenchman, who when he came to handle them, they would not endure him, but ran and hid

F 4   in

in their hole ; then would he take his Cittern and play upon it : They, hearring his Mufick, came all crawling to his feet, and began to climbe up him, till he gave over playing, then away they ran.

This recalls to my mind, what fome men of repute, and particularly the Learned *Kircherus*, relate concerning a great Fifh, in or about the Streights that fever *Sicily* from *Italy*, which is faid to be much affected with a peculiar kind of Tune, (harfh enough to Humane ears) by which the Mariners are wont to allure it to follow their veffels. And it may much ftrengthen the Conclufion maintained in this Chapter, if there be any certainty in the famous tradition, that the Lion is terrified and made to run away by the crowing of a Cock : I fay, *if*, becaufe though I doubt not but fome peculiar kinds of Sounds, as well as of other fenfible objects, may be particularly and exceedingly ungratefull to the Senfories of this or that peculiar kind of Animals, and confequently

to

to the ears of Lions; yet a late French Traveller into the *Levant* gives me cause much to question the matter of fact, affirming, that rowing along the brink of *Tigris* or *Euphrates*, (for I do not punctually remember which,) they were, for many hours in the night, terrified by Lions that attended them along the brink of the River, and would not at all be frighted by the frequent crowing of the Cocks that chanced to be in the passengers Boat. Of which unconcernedness of the Lions, our observing traveller took much more notice than the Lions appeared to do of the crowing of the Cocks. I might on this occasion say something of the received Tradition, that many sleeping persons will be more easily waked by being called upon by their own usual names, than by other names, though uttered with a louder voice. But this it may suffice to have mentioned; nor will I here insist on that more certain example of the operation of a Sound, which is as-

for-

forded by the starting of men or greater Animals, upon a surprizing, though not vehement, noise; though this oftentimes puts so many of the Spirits and Muscles into motion, that the whole bulk of the Animal is suddenly raised from the ground, which perhaps it could not be by the bare counterpoise of some hundreds of pounds : This, I say, I will not in this place insist on, because the *Phænomenon* seems to depend rather upon the loudness or acuteness of the sound, than upon any determinate modification of it, particularly relating to the *Animal* it self.

But the eminentest Instance of the efficacy of peculiarly modified Sounds upon disposed bodies, is afforded by what happens to those which are bit by a *Tarantula*. For though the bitten person will calmly hear divers other tunes, yet when a peculiarly congruous one comes to be plaid, it will set him a dancing with so much vigour as the spectators cannot but wonder at, and the dancing will some-

ſometimes continue many hours, if the Muſick do ſo, and not otherwiſe. I know there are ſome that queſtion the truth of the things related of theſe *Tarantati,* (as the *Italians* call them,)and I eaſily grant,that ſome Fictions may have been ſuffered to paſs under the countenance of ſo ſtrange a Truth. But beſides the affirmations of ſome Learned men, (as well Phyſicians as others) my Doubts have been much removed by the Accounts I have received from an Ingenious Acquaintance of mine own,who at *Tarentum* it ſelf, whence the Inſect takes its name, and elſewhere,ſaw many bitten perſons in their dances,ſome in publick and ſome in private places, and amongſt the reſt a Phyſician, on whom the tune that fitted his diſtemper had the ſame operation as on the other Patients. And the Learned *Epiphanius Ferdinandus*, who practiſed Phyſick in *Apulia* and *Calabria* for many years, not onely delivers upon his own perſonal obſervation, ſeveral Narratives of the effects

effects of Mufick upon the *Tarantati*, but invites any that may doubt of the truth of fuch Narratives to repair to him at a fit feafon, undertaking to convince them by ocular Demonftration.

I know a very honeft and fober Mufician, who has divers times affirmed to me, that he could at pleafure, by playing a certain Tune, (which he acquainted me with, and which did not much move others) make a perfon (whom he named to me) weep, whether fhe would or no. And I might add, that when I have been taking Phyfick, or am any thing feverifh, the repetition of two verfes of *Lucan* feldom fails (as I have often tried) of producing in me a chilnefs, almoft like that, but fainter, that begins the fit of an ague. But on this Inftance I look not as a ftrong proof of the Phyfical efficacy of Sounds; becaufe thofe two verfes having been emphatically read, when divers years agoe I lay fick of a flow fever, and could not reft, they made

so

fo ftrong an impreffion on me, that whenever I am under a Difcompo-fure any thing near like that, that then troubled me, thofe verfes re-vive, as 'twere, in my brain and fome other parts that difpofition, or ra-ther indifpofition, with which my firft hearing of thofe verfes was ac-companied.

It may be the lefs admired, that the vibrating motion of the Air, that produces founds, fhould have fuch effects upon difpofed Organical bo-dies, fince Light it felf, which ei-ther confilts of briskly moving *ef-fluvia* far more fubtile than aerial corpufcles, or is propagated by the pulfe of a far more fubtile body than Air, may have a notable ope-ration upon difpofed bodies. For we commonly obferve, that the Sun-beams, by beating upon the face or eyes of fome that come fuddenly out of a fhaded place into the Light, prefently make them fneeze; which you know is not done without a ve-hement motion of divers parts of the

the body. And though Colour be but
a modification of Light; yet, besides
that 'twas anciently a practice, as the
History of the *Macchabees* informs
us, to shew red objects to Elephants,
to make them more fierce, 'tis a fa-
miliar observation, that red cloaths
do offend and irritate Turky-cocks.
And that is more remarkable, which
is related by the very Learned Physi-
cian *Valesius*, of a person that he knew,
who, if he looked upon red objects,
would not onely have his Eyes offended, but was subject to an effusion
of Humours in the neighboring parts.

CHAP.

CHAP. VII.

Obſervat. VI. Men ſuſpect not what efficacy the Inviſible motions of Fluids may have, even upon inorganical bodies, upon the ſcore of ſome determinate Congruity or relation betwixt a peculiar Texture of the one, and the peculiar modification of the others motion.

Though the Experiments delivered in the foregoing Chapter have, I preſume, ſufficiently manifeſted, that the modification given to the motions of the Air by ſonorous bodies may have conſiderable effects upon Animals, in whoſe organized bodies the curiouſly contrived parts have an admirable connexion with, and relation to, one another, and to the whole Symmetrical fabrick they make up; yet, I fear, it will ſcarce ſeem credible, that ſonorous motions of the Air, not very loud, ſhould find, even in

bodies

bodies Inanimate and Inorganicall, such congruous Textures and other Difpofitions to admit their action, that even more languid Sounds, peculiarly modified, may fenfibly operate upon them, and much more than founds that are louder and more vehement, but not fo happily modified. To make this good by particular Experiments, I fhall begin with that, which, though the effect may feem inferiour to that of moft of the others, I judge fitteft to manifeft, that the produced motion depends upon the determinate modification of that of the impellent Fluid.

That a certain impulfe of Air, made by one of the Unifon-ftrings of a Mufical Inftrument, may fuffice to produce a vifible motion in another, is now become a known experiment; of the Caufe and fome unobferved Phænomena of which I elfewhere more fully difcourfe. But, that it may not be fufpected in this cafe, that the fhake of the untouched ftring is communicated to it by the

propa-

propagated motion of the Inſtrument it ſelf, to which the ſtring, that is ſtruck, is alſo faſtned; I ſhall add, that, according to what I elſewhere relate, I found by trial purpoſely made; that a ſtring of Wire, (which you will grant to be a more ſolid body than an ordinary Gut-ſtring,) may be without another ſtring brought to tremble by a determinate Sound made at a diſtance, which produced but ſuch an impulſe of the Air, as could neither be ſeen nor felt by the By-ſtanders, nor would communicate any ſenſible motion to the neighbouring ſtrings. 'Tis true, that in this caſe the ſtring, in which the trembling was produced, was a ſingle, long, ſlender and ſpringy body, faſtned at both ends to a ſtable one; and therefore it may ſeem altogether groundleſs to expect, that any thing like this effect ſhould be by the ſame cauſe produced in bodies that do not appear ſo qualified. But, as we elſewhere ſhew, that a certain degree or meaſure of tenſion is in or-

G   der

der to this Phænomenon the principal Qualification, without which all the other would be unavailable; perhaps 'twill not be abfurd to enquire, *whether*, in bodies of a very differing appearance from ftrings, the various Textures, Connexions, and Complications, that Nature or Art, or both, may make of the parts, may not bring them to a ftate equivalent to the Tenfions of the ftrings of Mufical Inftruments, whereby divers of the mentioned parts may be ftretched in the manner requifite to difpofe them to receive a vibrating motion from fome peculiar Sounds: And *whether* thefe trembling parts may not be numerous enough to affect their neighbours, and make, in the body they belong to, a tremulous motion difcernible, though not by the Eye, yet by fome other fenfe. This conjecture or inquiry you will, I hope, have the lefs unfavourable thoughts of, when you fhall have confidered the following Experiments.

I remember, that many years agoe
I found

I found by trial, that, if a somewhat large and almost hemispherical Glasse, though not very thin, were conveniently placed, a determinate sound, made at a convenient distance from the concave surface of the Glasse, would make it sensibly ring, as a Bell does a while after it has been struck. But this noise was the effect of a determinate sound; for, though the voice were raised to a higher tone, or if the sound were made louder, the same effect would not insue. I remember also, that, some years after, I observed, that large empty drinking-glasses of fine white metal had each of them its determinate Tension, or some disposition that was equivalent as to our purpose. For, causing the strings of a Musical Instrument to be variously screwed up, and let down, and briskly struck, we found, as I expected, that the motion of one string, when 'twas stretched to a certain note or tone, would make one of the Glasses ring, and not the other; nor would the sound of the

G 2　　　　same

fame ftring, tuned to another note, fenfibly affect the firft Glaffe, though perhaps it might have its operation upon another. And this Circum-ftance is not, on this occafion, to be omitted, that, after we had found the tone proper to one of the Glaffes, and fo tuned the ftring, that, (I fay) when that was ftruck, the Glaffe would refound. Having afterwards broken off a part of the foot of the glafs, yet not fo much but that it con-tinued to ftand upright, the fame found of the ftring would no longer be anfwered by the Veffel, but we were obliged to alter the tenfion of the ftring, to produce the former ef-fect. The Learned *Kircherus*, as I have been informed, fomewhere mentions a correfpondence between fome li-quours and fome determinate founds; which I fuppofe may be true, though the triall did not fucceed with me, perhaps for want of fuch accommo-dations for fo nice an Experiment as I could have wifhed, but could not procure: But if you can, you will ob-
lige

lige me to make the trials fo as to fa-
tisfie your felf and me, whether the
agitation of the liquour be caufed immediately by the motion of the Air,
or be communicated by the interven-
tion of the tremblings of the Veffel.

An Artift famous for his skill in
making Organs, anfwered me, that,
at fome ftops of the Organs, fome
feats in the Church would tremble.
But, becaufe I fufpected by his Relation, that the greatnefs of the found
chiefly effected it, becaufe, when
that Pipe, which they call the open
Diapafon, founds, the chair or feat,
on which the Organift fits, and perhaps the neighbouring part of the
Organ trembles ; I fhall add, that I
have divers times obferved certain
founds of an excellent Organ to make
not onely the feat, I fate on in the
Church, tremble under me, but produce an odd tremulous motion in the
upper part of my Hat, that I could
plainly feel with my hands.   And
that, which makes me apt to believe
that this effect depends upon the de-

ᵗerminate tone, rather than upon the
ˡoudneſs of the ſound, is, that I have
oftentimes felt, and diligently obſerved ſuch a kind of motion in the upper part of my Hat, upon the pro-
nouncing of ſome words in ordinary
diſcourſe; in which caſe the effect
could not with probability be referred to the greatneſs of the Sound, but
its peculiar fitneſs to communicate
ſuch a motion to a body ſo diſpoſed.

Nor is it onely in ſuch ſmall and
yielding bodies, as Hats and Strings,
that Sounds that are not boiſterous
may produce ſenſible effects, for, if
they be congruous to the Texture
of the body they are to work on,
they may excite motions in it, though
it be either ſolid or very bulky: of
which I ſhall here ſubjoyn a couple
of inſtances.

An ancient Muſician affirmed to
me, that, playing on a Baſe-viol in the
chamber of one of his Scholars, when
he came to ſtrike a certain Note on
a particular ſtring, he heard an odd
kind of jarring Noiſe, which he
thought

thought at firſt had either been caſu-
al, or proceeded from ſome fault
in the ſtring; but, having afterwards
frequent occaſion to play in that ſame
room, he plainly found, that the
Noiſe, he marvelled at, was made by
the tremulous motion of a Caſement
of a window, which would be made
to tremble by a determinate ſound
of a particular ſtring, and not by o-
ther Notes, whether higher or lower.

To this firſt Inſtance I ſhall add the
ſecond, which, I confeſſe, I was not
forward to believe, till trial had con-
vinced me of the Truth; and I ſcru-
pled it the rather, becauſe, if the re-
flexion of determinate Sounds ſhould
appear to proceed from the peculiar
kind of tremulous motion into which
the parts of the reſonant body are
put, it may incline men to ſo great
a Paradox, as to think, that ſuch a
motion of the Air as our Bodies do
not feel, may produce a trembling in
ſo ſolid a body as a Stone-wall of a
great thickneſs. The Experiment or
Obſervation it ſelf I ſhall give you

in the same words I set it down some hours after I made it, which were these.

Yesterday I went to satisfy my self of the truth of what had been told me by an ancient Musician, to whom I had been relating what I had observed of the effects of some determinate Sounds even upon Solid bodies, and of whom I enquired, if he had met with any thing of the like nature : taking him along with me, I found, that though the place be but an Arch, yet it would not answer to all notes indifferently, when we stood in a certain place, but to a determinate Note, (which he afterwards told me was *Ce fa ut* a little flatted,) to which note it answered very resonantly, and not sensibly to others, which we made trial of, whether higher or lower than it ; and, (which added to the strangeness,) when I made him raise his voice to an Eighth, as consonant as those two Sounds are wont to be in all other cases, the vaulted Arch did not appear

pear to us affected with the Note. The Musician added, that he had tried in most Arches all about the City, and could not find such a peculiarity in them, as being to be made resonant by all Notes or Sounds indifferently that were strong enough; and also, that as this Arch for this hundred years has been observed to have this property, so an ancient and experienced Builder informed him, that any Vault that were exquisitely built, would peculiarly answer to some determinate Note or other.

CHAP.

CHAP. VIII.

Obfervat. VII. Men look upon divers Bodies as having their parts in a ftate of abfolute Reft, when indeed they are in a Forced ftate, as of Tenfion, Compreffion, &c.

THis Obfervation will probably feem paradoxicall. For, when an intire Body, efpecially if it be of a folid Confiftence, and feem to be of an homogeneous or uniform matter, appears to be moveleffe, we are wont to take it for granted, that the parts, which that body is made up of, are perfectly at Reft alfo. But yet this will fcarce be thought a reafonable fuppofition, if we do but rightly confider fome obvious *Phænomena,* which may teach us, that, whilft a whole Body, or the fuperficies that includes it, retains its figure, dimenfions and diftance from other ftable Bodies that are near it, the Corpufcles that compofe it may have

various

various and brisk motions and endea-
vours among themselves. As, when
a bar of iron or silver, having been
well hammered, is newly taken off of
the Anvill; though the Eye can
discern no motion in it, yet the touch
will readily perceive it to be very
hot, and, if you spit upon it, the
brisk agitation of the insensible parts
will become visible in that which
they will produce in the liquour. Besides, when the Lath of a Crofs-bow
stands bent, though a man do neither by the Eye nor the Touch perceive any motion in the springy parts,
yet if the string be cut or broken,
the sudden and vehement motion of
the Lath, tending to restore it to the
figure it had before it was bent, dif-
covers a springinefs; whence we
conclude it was before in a state of
violent Compreffion. And, though
the string of a bent Bow do like-
wife appear to be in a state of Reft;
yet, if you cut it afunder, the newly
made extreams will fly from one another suddenly and forcibly enough

to

to manifeſt, that they were before in
a violent ſtate of Tenſion.   And on
this occaſion I could add divers Inſtances taken not onely from the
works of Art, but thoſe of Nature
too, if they did not belong to another paper : But, one ſort of Obſervations 'twill be proper to ſet down
in this place ; becauſe in thoſe already mentioned, the bow and ſtring
were brought into a violent ſtate by
the meer and immediate force of
man.   I ſhall therefore add, that
there are divers bodies, in which,
though no ſuch kind of force appears
to have antecedently acted on them,
we may yet take notice of a ſtate of
violent Compreſſion or Extenſion,
and a ſtrong endeavour or tendency
of the parts, that to the Eye or the
Touch ſeem at reſt, to ſhrink or to
fly out ; and this endeavour may in
ſome Caſes be more laſting and more
forcible than one would eaſily ſuſpect
or believe.   But examples of this
kind you muſt not expect that I
ſhould give you out of *Claſſick* Au-
thours,

thours, since in them 'tis like you
have not met with either an Instance
or a Conjecture to this purpose; but
some few things that I tried my self,
and some others that I learnt by
Inquiry from some Tradesmen,
whom I judged likeliest to inform
me, I shall briefly acquaint you
with.

I have sometimes observed my
self, and have had the Observation
confirmed to me by the ingeniouser
Traders in Glass; That a Glass, that
seemed to have been well baked,
or nealed, (as they call it) would sometimes, many days or weeks, or perhaps months, after it is taken from the
fire, crack of its own accord; which
seems for the most part to happen
upon the score of the strong, but un-
equall, shrinking of the parts of the
Glasse. And the Glass-men will tell
you, that, if they take their Glasses
too hastily from the fire, not allowing
them leisure to cool by degrees,
they will be very apt to crack. But
I remember, that, to satisfy some Ingenious

genious men, I devifed a way of ex-
hibiting a much more quick and remarkable *Phænomenon* of that kind.
Having made then, by a way I elfewhere teach, a flat Lump of metalline Glafs, two or three or four times
as thick as an ordinary Drinking-
glafs, I obferved, as I expected, that,
though it had been melted in a very
gentle fire, its very fufible nature
needing no other, and though it were
removed but very little from the fire,
it was fo difpofed to fhrink upon
a fmall degree of Refrigeration, or
rather abatement of Heat, that, before it was fenfibly cold, it would
crack with a noife in fo vehement a
manner, that, notwithftanding the
ponderoufnefs of the matter, which
had been purpofely laid upon a Le-
vell, parts of a confiderable bulk,
weighing perhaps fome Drams,
would fly, to a not inconfiderable
diftance from one another. And
this Experiment I took pleafure to
make more than once. And if you
will be content with an Inftance
which,

which, though otherwife much inferiour, may not be unwelcome, for
its being eafily and readily made; I
fhall offer you one that I have often
repeated. Take a piece of Copper,
(if the Plate be thick, 'tis fo much
the better,) and, having throughly
brought it to a red or white Heat
among kindled Coals, take it from
the fire, and when it begins to cool
a little, hold it over a fheet or two
of white Paper, and you will perceive good ftore of flakes to fly off,
not without fome little noife, one after the other, and fometimes perhaps
as far as the farthermoft edges of the
paper; which flakes or fcales feem
by their brittlenefs and colour, to
be but parts of the furface of the metal vitrified by the vehement action
of the fire, and afterwards by a too
hafty refrigeration fhrinking fo violently, as to crack and leap from
one another, like the contiguous
parts of the ftring of a Viol or other
Mufical Inftrument, that breaks by
the moifture of the Air. And on
this

this occasion I shall add, that, having afterwards inquired of an expert Artificer, that made metalline Concaves, about the shrinking of his mixtures of metalls, he confessed to me, that he usually observed them to shrink upon Refrigeration.   And the like I my self have observed in Iron of a great thickness, and purposely fitted to a hollow body of metall, which it would not enter when it was ignited, though it would when 'twas cold. But to shew you by a notable Instance or two, both that Metals may shrink, and that they may doe so with a very considerable force, I shall add, that I found by inquiry, that the lately mentioned Artificer, after he had made some large Concaves of an unfit mixture of metals, and having removed them from the fire, had been very carefull to keep the cold Air from them, lest they should cool too hastily, observed yet to his great loss, that, when they came to be further refrigerated, they would (perhaps after three hours) crack with a great noise,

though

though this metalline mixture were perchance harder than Iron, and three or four times as thick as common Looking-glasses. But the misfortune of another Tradesman afforded me a yet more considerable *Phænomenon.* For this excellent Artificer, whom I often employ, and with whom I was a while since discoursing of these matters, complain'd to me, that, having lately cast a kind of Bell-metall upon a very strong solid Instrument of Iron of a considerable superficial *Area,* though the metal were suffer'd in a warm room to cool, from about eight a clock on Saturday night till about ten or twelve on Monday morning, and were then (which is to be noted) considerably hot to the touch; yet it cool'd so far, that, shrinking from the Iron that would not shrink with it, the Bell-metall cracked in divers places with noises loud as the Report of a Pistoll, though the metall, he affirm'd to me, was an inch and half, or two inches thick. And the same

H   person

person shewed me a large Cylinder of Iron, about which, for a certain purpose, a Coat of Bell-metall had been cast some days before, on which (Bell-metall) there was a crack near one end made by the coldness of the Iron, though the thickness of the Bell-metall, as near as I could measure it, exceeded an inch, and (as the Workman affirmed) an inch and a quarter.

Nor is it onely in such mixtures as Bell-metall, which, though very hard, may be very brittle, but even in a metal that is malleable when cold, that the like Phænomenon may be met with, as I have been assured by another ingenious Artificer, of whom I inquired, whether he had taken notice of the shrinking of metalls; who affirm'd to me, that, having had occasion to cast about a Cylinder of Iron a ring or hoop of Brass, he found to his trouble, that, when the metall began to cool, the parts shrunk from one another so as to leave a gaping crack, which he was fain to

fill

fill up with ſoulder quite croſſe the breadth of the ring, though this were above an inch thick.

I ſhould not, *Pyrophilus*, have in this Chapter entertained you with more Experiments of others than of my own, if I had the conveniency of living near Founders of metalls, as the Tradeſmen had whoſe Obſervations I have recited, and whoſe ſincerity in them I had no cauſe to queſtion. And both their Experiments and mine ſeem to teach, that a body may be brought into a ſtate of Tenſion, as well by being expanded and ſtretch'd by the action of the fire upon the minute parts, as by the action of an external Agent upon the intire body. And, to ſpeak more generally, the ſtate of violent Contraction and Compreſſion may not unfitly be illuſtrated by a Bow that is bent. For, as the Bow it ſelf is brought to a ſtate of Compreſſion by the force of the Archer, that bent it; ſo by the Elaſtical force of the bent Bow, the ſtring is brought into a violent ſtate

H 2　　　　　of

of Tenſion, as may be made evident
by the cutting off the ſtring in the
middle; for then both the Bow will
fly ſuddenly outwards, and the parts
of the ſtring will ſwiftly and violently ſhrink from one another. And
according to this Doctrine, the effect
of other bodies upon ſuch as are thus
brought into, what men call, a Preternatural ſtate, is not to be judg'd
barely according to uſual meaſures,
but with reſpect to this latent Diſpo-
ſition of the Patient : as, for inſtance,
though the ſtring of a Viol not ſcrew-
ed up, will not be hardned by the
vapours that imbue the Air in moiſt
weather; yet a neighbouring ſtring
of the ſame Inſtrument, though perhaps much ſtronger, being ſcrew'd
up, and thereby ſtretched, will be ſo
affected with thoſe vapours, as to
break with noiſe and violence. And
ſo when one part of a piece of Glaſs
is made as hot as can be, without
appearing diſcolour'd to the Eye,
though a drop or two of cold water
have no effect upon the other part of
the

the same Glasse, yet if it touch the
heated part, whose wonted extension
(as I have elsewhere proved) is alter'd by the fire that vehemently
agitates the component particles, the
cracking of the Glass will almost always presently ensue.

If against these Instances it be alledged, that it is possible to assign another cause of the seemingly sponta-
neous breaking of the bodies mention'd in this Chapter, than that
which I have propos'd, it will not
much concern this Discourse to ex-
amine the Allegation; for, whatever
the latent Cause of the Phænomena
may be, the manifest Circumstances of
them suffice to shew, that bodies,
which, as to sense, are in a natural
state of Rest, may be in a violent
one, as of Tension, and may have,
either upon the score of the contex-
ture of the parts among themselves,
or upon that of some interfluent subtile matter, or some other Physical
Agent, a strong endeavour to fly off
or recede from one another; and that,

H 3   in

in divers bodies, the caufe of this endeavour may act more vigoroufly
than one would eafily believe: and
this fuffices to ferve the turn of this
Difcourfe. For I prefume that a
perfon of your Principles will allow,
that Local Motion muft be produc'd
by Local Motion, and confequently,
that, without a very ftrong, though
invifible and unheeded one, fuch hard
and folid bodies as thick pieces of
metall could not be made to crack.

I know not whether I may on this
occafion acquaint you with an odd
Relation I had from a very honeft
and credible, as well as experienced,
Artift, whom I, for thofe reafons,
have feveral times made choice to
deal with about precious Stones, and
other things belonging to the Jewel-
lers and Goldfmiths trades. For,
confidering with him one day a large
lump of matter, which contained feveral Stones that he took for courfe
Agats, and which were joyned together by a Cement, that in moft
places was harder than moft ordinary

ry Stones, I perceived that there remained divers pretty large cavities in this Cement, which seemed to have contained such Stones as those that yet made parts of the lump. Upon which occasion he affirmed to me, that several of the Stones grew whilst they were lodg'd in those cavities. And when I told him, that, though I had been long of an opinion, that Stones may receive an increment after their first formation, yet I did not see how any such thing appeared by those we were looking upon : He gave me in many words an account of his Assertion, which I reduced to this, that the Stones he spoke of, did, after they were first formed, really tend to expand themselves by virtue of some Principle of growth, which he could not intelligibly describe ; but that these Stones being lodg'd in a Cement extreamly hard, and therefore not capable of being forced to give way, their expansive endeavour was rendered ineffectual, but not destroyed : so that when afterwards these

Stones

Stones came to be taken out of the Cement wherein they were bedded, and to whofe fides 'tis like they were not exquifitely congruous, the compreft Stones, having their fides now no longer wedged in by the harder Cement, quickly expanded themfelves, as if 'twere by an internal and violently compreft fpring, and would prefently burft afunder, fome into two, and fome into more pieces: of which he prefented many to his friends, but yet had referved fome, whereof he prefented me one, that I have yet by me, together with fome of the mafs, whofe Cement I find to bear a better polifh than marble, and to be very much harder than it. And, in anfwer to fome queftions of mine, he told me, that he had taken up thefe Stones himfelf, naming the place to me, which was not very far off, and that he obferved all that he told me himfelf, and more than once or twice, and that I needed not fufpect, as I feemed to doe, that 'twas the ftrokes employed to force the

Stones

Stones out of their Beds, that made them break. For, besides that many of them, which (it seems) were not compreſt enough, did not break, ſeveral of thoſe, that did, were taken out, without offering them any ſuch violence, as that their burſting could with any probability be imputed to it.

CHAP.

CHAP. IX.

Observat. VIII. *One main cause why such Motions as we speak of are over-look'd, is, That we are scarce wont to take notice but of those motions of Solid bodies, wherein one whole Body drives away another, or at least knocks visibly against it, whereas many effects proceed from the intestine motions produced by the external Agent, in, and among, the parts of the same body.*

THis Observation is like to be much more readily understood than granted, and therefore I shall offer by way of proof the following Experiments.

We caused in a large brass Stop-cock the movable part to be nimbly turned to and fro in the contiguous cavity of that part that was made to receive it, in that part of the Instrument that is wont to be kept fixt. And though this motion of the Key

were

were made onely by the bare hand,
yet in a short time the mutual attrition of the contiguous parts of the
Instrument made so brisk an agitation in the other parts, that the inca-
lescence made the metal it self to
swell, insomuch that the Key could
no more be turned, but remained fixt,
as if it had been wedged in, so that,
to make it work as before, it was
necessary by cooling it to make it
shrink a little, and so take off the
mutual pressure of the Key, and the
other part of the Stop-cock. Nor is
this to be looked on as a casual Experiment; for, besides that it was
made more than once, and is very
analogous to some other trials of
mine; I found, that a maker of such
Instruments complained to me, that
he was several times forced to inter-
mit his work, and plunge his Instrument in cold water, before he could,
by grinding, adjust the Key to the
cavity it ought to fit.

I presume I need not take notice
to you, that this Experiment confirms
what

what I elsewhere mention of the dilatation of metals themselves by Heat, and therefore I proceed to the next Instance.

This is afforded by the known Experiment of passing one's wetted finger upon the orifice of a Drinking-glass almost fill'd with water. For, though the Eye does not immediately discern any motion, that, by reason of the pressure of the finger, is made by one part of the glass upon another ; yet, That a vibrating motion is thereby produced, may be argued by the dancing of the water, especially that which is contiguous to the prest sides of the glass, by which 'tis oftentimes so agitated, that numerous drops are made to leap quite over, and others are tossed up to a good height into the Air. And that there may be considerable motions in the sides of the glass, whilst it does not break in pieces, we may probably guess by this, that, in Drinking-glasses artificially cut by a spiral line, both I, and others, have

often

often found by trial, that, a glass
being dextrously inverted and shaken, the parts will vibrate up and
down so manifestly, as sometimes to
lengthen the glass, by my estimate,
a quarter of an inch or more, and
yet, the glass being set again upon
its foot, it appeared that it had not
been hereby at all injured.

That two pieces of Iron or Steel,
by being strongly rubbed against one
another, will at length acquire a temporary Heat, is not hard to be belie-
ved: but that an edg'd Tool of hardened Steel should, by having its
edge rubbed against, have a manifest
and permanent change made in its
Texture, you did not perhaps suspect;
and yet, having had the Curiosity to
cause some metals, and particularly
Iron and Steel, to be turned by an
excellent Artificer, I learned partly
by his experience, and partly by my
own, that the edge of the Steel-tool,
with which he by degrees shaved off
the protuberant parts of the metal,
would be so heated and agitated,
that,

that, in no long time, if care were not
taken to prevent it, the tool would
be brought to look of blewish and
yellowish colours, and, permanently
losing its former temper, would become so soft, as to be uselesse for its
former work, unlesse it were again
artificially hardened : and therefore,
to prevent the trouble of tempering
his tools again, this Artist, from time
to time, dipt it, when it began to
grow too hot, into a certain liquour,
which he affirms, upon much experience, to have a peculiar fitness for that
purpose.

Nor is it always necessary that the
body, that makes the parts of an
inanimate body work considerably
on one another, should be either
very hard, or impetuously moved.
For, I remember, that, having once
by me some short bars of fine Tin, I
resolved to try whether, meerly with
my naked hands, (which you know
are none of the strongest or hardest,)
I could not procure a considerable
internal Commotion among the parts;
and

and accordingly, laying hold on the two ends of the bar with my two hands, I flowly bent the bar towards me and from me two or three times, and having by this means broke or cracked it in the midft, I perceived, as I expected, that the middle parts had confiderably heated each other.

What ufe may be made of this Experiment in the fearch of the hidden caufe of Elafticity, would be lefs properly confidered in this place than in another. But fince I have named that Quality, I fhall take this rife to intimate, that if the reftitution of a fpringy body, forcibly bent, proceed onely (as fome Learned Moderns would have it) from the endeavour of the compreft parts themfelves to recover their former ftate, one may not impertinently take notice of the Elafticity that Iron, Silver and Brafs acquire by hammering, among the Inftances that fhew what in fome cafes may be done by a motion wherein the parts of the fame body are, by

ap

an almost unheeded force, put to act upon one another. But if Springiness depend chiefly upon the pervasion of a subtile matter, as the *Cartesians* would have it, then the Instances will properly belong to another Subject.

§ The foregoing Examples may also suffice to make out (what I am unwilling to refer to another Head) this subordinate Observation, That men are more usually than justly prepossessed with an opinion, that nothing considerable is to be expected from the motion of a body against another, unless the former do make a manifest percussion or trusion of the latter. But, because this prepossession especially prevails in cases where the body that is by friction or attrition to affect the other, is it self soft or yielding, I shall on this occasion add a few Instances to remove this Prejudice.

An Artist, eminent for grinding of Optical glasses, confessed to me, that sometimes when he went about

to

to polish his broader glasses, though but upon a piece of Leather sprinkled with Puttee, that friction did so heat or otherwise agitate the parts of the glass, as, to his great loss, to make it crack from the edge to the middle; which seemed the more strange, because we see, what intense degrees of Heat glasses will endure without cracking, if the fire be but gradually applied, as this Artist's glasses must have been gradually heated.

But I think it worth inquiry, whether in this case the whole work be performed by meer Heat, and whether there intervene not a peculiar kind of motion, into which some bodies are disposed to be put by a peculiar kind of friction, which seems fitted to produce in manifestly springy bodies, and perhaps in some others, (of which divers may be springy that are not commonly taken to be so,) such a vibrating or reciprocal motion, as may have some notable effects, that are not wont to be produced by

I   mode-

moderate Heats, nor always by intenfe ones themfelves. The trembling of the parts of a Drinking-glafs, and the vifible vibration of the long and great ftrings of a Bafe-viol, upon peculiar founds, may give fome countenance to this conjecture. And that in fome bodies there may be fuch a tremulous motion produced, by rubbing them upon fo foft a thing as Wool, or upon a piece of Cloath, I tried by this Experiment :

We caft into a hollow Veffel, very fmooth within, and of an almoft Hemifpherical figure, feverall ounces of good melted Brimftone, and having fuffered it to cool, and taken it out, the Convex furface, as had been defired, came off well polifhed; then this conveniently fhaped lump, which had (if I well remember) four or five inches in Diameter, being briskly rubbed in the fame line forwards and backwards, upon a Cufhion or fome fuch woollen thing, in a place free from other noifes, I could, by holding my ear to it, and attentively liftening,

ftening, plainly hear a crackling noife made by the agitated parts, which continued a brisk, and, as I fuppofed, a vibrating motion for fome time after the friction was ended.

That there may be a confiderable Commotion produced among the internal parts of bodies, by rubbing them even againft foft bodies, I have divers times obferved, by the fulphureous fteams that I could fmell, if, after having a little rubbed a lump of good Sulphur upon my Cloaths, I prefently held it to my nofe. Which brings into my mind, that I have had the like effect from much harder and clofer bodies than Sulphur, when they were rubbed upon bodies that were fo too. For having purpofely taken hard Stones cut out of mens Bladders, and rubbed a couple of them a little againft one another, they quickly afforded, as I expected, a rank fmell of ftale Urin.

That Diamonds themfelves will, by rubbing upon woollen cloaths, be made Electrical, feems to argue, that

I 2   even

even Their parts are set a moving:
And that the Commotion reaches to
the internal parts, I am the more
apt to think, because I have a Diamond, that, if I rub it well and
luckily against my Cloaths, will, for
a little while, shine or glimmer in
the dark; which is the same Phænomenon that I elsewhere relate my
self to have produced in the King's
larger Diamond, by giving it one brisk
stroke with the point of a bodkin,
where the Light that presently appeared in the Gem, seemed not re-
ferrable to any thing so likely as the
sudden Commotion made in the internal parts of that peculiarly consti-
tuted Stone.

What a peculiar modification of
motion, distinct from its degrees of
Impetus, may doe in Fluid bodies, we
have formerly in this Essay taken notice of. But perhaps it may be
worth while to enquire, what kinds
there are of it, and what effects they
may have in the parts of Solid bodies themselves. For I have obser-

ved,

ved, that though thofe Stones that the *Italian* Glafs-men ufe are very hard, and, if I mifremember not, have feveral times afforded me fparks of fire by Collifion ; yet, by rubbing them a little one againft another, I found, that fuch an agitation was made in their parts, as to make them throw out ftore of fœtid exhalations: And 'tis poffibly to the ftony Ingredient that Glafs owes the Quality I have obferved in it, and elfewhere mentioned, of emitting offenfive fteams. And 'tis remarkable to our prefent purpofe, that, though fo vehement an agitation of the parts, as is given to Glafs by Heat, when 'tis made almoft red-hot in the fire, does not make it fenfibly emit odours ; yet barely by dextroufly rubbing two folid pieces of Glafs againft one another, one may, in a minute of an hour, make thofe fixed bodies emit fuch copious fteams as I found, not onely fenfibly, but rankly, fœtid; though one would think thofe ftinking exhalations very indifpofed to be forced off, fince they

were

were not expelled by the vehement
fire, that the Glaſs long endured
in the furnace where 'twas kept melted.

There are few things that ſhew
better, both how the parts of Inorganical bodies communicate their vibrating motions to one another, and
how brisk thoſe motions are, than
that which happens upon the ſtriking
of a large Bell with a Clapper or a
Hammer.   For though the ſtroak be
immediately made but upon one part;
yet the motion, thereby produced,
is propagated to the oppoſite, and
the ſucceſſive vibrations of the ſmall
parts do, even in ſo ſolid and cloſe
a body as Bell-metal, run many times
round ; as may appear by the dura-
bleneſs of the ringing noiſe, which
ſeems plainly to proceed from the
circularly ſucceſſive vibrations of
the parts, which, unleſs they briskly
tremble themſelves, can ſcarcely be
conceived to be fitted to give the
Air that tremulous motion, whoſe
effect on the Ear, when the firſt and
loud

loud noise, made by the percuſſion, is paſt, we call Ringing. And this mo-tion of the parts of the ſounding Bell may be further argued by this, that, if the finger, or ſome other ſoft body, be laid upon it, the ſound will be checked or deaded, and much more, if a broad ſtring, though of a ſoft ſubſtance, be tied about it. And not onely an attentive Ear may of-ten make us gueſs, that the ringing ſound is produced by a motion pro-pagated circularly in the Bell, but this vibrating motion may ſometimes be alſo felt by the tremulous motion communicated by the trembling parts of the Bell to the finger, that is wari-ly applied to it. That this motion paſſes in a round, from one ſide of the Bell to the other, ſeems manifeſt by the great difference of ſound, e-ſpecially in regard of ringing, that may be obſerved in a ſound Bell, and in a crack'd one ; where yet all the matter and the former figure are pre-ſerved, onely the intireneſs or conti-nuity, which is neceſſary to the circu-

lation

lation (if I may so call it) of the tremulous motion, is at the Crack stopt or hindred. And that the motion of the parts is very brisk, may be guessed partly by what has been said already; but much more if that be true, which, not onely is traditionally reported by many, but has been affirmed to me by several Artificers that deal in Bells, who averred, as an experienced thing, That if a conveniently sized Bell were bound about, any thing hard, with a broad string, and then struck with the usual force, that it would otherwise bear very well; that percussion would break it, giving a disorderly check to the brisk motion of the parts of the Bell, whereof some happening to be much more (and otherwise) agitated than others, the force of their motion surmounts that of their Cohesion, and so produces a Crack.

But, in regard great Bells are not easie to be procured, nor to be managed when one has accesse to them, I shall add, that I took the Bell of a

large

large Watch, or very small Clock made of fine Bell-metall, which had no handle or other thing put to it, save a little Bodkin or skiver of wood, whose point we thrust into the hole that is usually left in the middle of the *Basis*; and this sharp piece of wood serving for a handle to keep the Bell steady enough, we placed in the cavity of it, near the edges, (for that Circumstance must not be omitted,) some black mineral Sand, or, in want of that, some small filings of Steel or Copper, or some other such minute and solid Powder, which yet must not be too small, and then striking moderately with the Key against the side of the Bell, we observed, (as we expected) that, whilst it continued briskly ringing, it made many of the filings to dance up and down, and sometimes to leap up, almost like the drops of Water, formerly mentioned to skip, when the brim of the Glass was circularly prest by the wetted finger. Which prompts me to add, that, having put a middle-
sized

fized drop of water (for in this cafe
the quantity is a confiderable Cir-
cumftance) near the lower edge of
the Bell, 'twas eafie to make it vifibly
tremble, and be as it were covered
over with little waves, by a fomewhat brisk ftroke of the Key on the
oppofite fide.   And this effect was
more confpicuous, when a very large
drop of water was placed near the
edge, on the convex fide of a hand-
Bell, whofe Clapper was kept from
any where touching the infide of it.
And to obviate their jealoufie, that,
not having feen the manner of the
above-mentioned motion of the Sand,
might fufpect that 'twas produced by
the impulfe which the Bell, as an intire body, received from the percuffion made by the Key, we feveral
times forbare putting-in the filings,
till after the ftroke had been given;
which fatisfied the Spectatours, that
the dancing and leaping of the minute bodies proceeded from the fame
brisk vibrations of the fmall parts
of the Bell, which, at the fame time
striking

striking also the Air, produced a ringing found, which might very well, as it did, out-last the skipping of the filings; the exceedingly minute particles of the Air being much more easily agitable, than the comparatively grofs and heavy Corpufcles of the Powder. And this fuccefs our Experiment had in a Bell, that little exceeded an inch and half in Diameter.

And here, *Pyroph.* I fhall put an end to this Rhapfody of Obfervations, hoping, that, among fo many of them, fome or other will be able to engage you, if not to conclude, yet at leaft to fufpect, that fuch Local motions, as are wont either to be paft-by unobferved, or be thought not worth the obferving, may have a notable operation, though not upon the generality of bodies, yet upon fuch as are peculiarly difpofed to admit it, and fo may have a confiderable fhare in the production of divers difficult *Phænomena* of nature, that are wont to be referred to lefs genuine, as well as lefs intelligible, Caufes.

FINIS.

9 781171 283188